LISTEN

AND

LOSE WEIGHT

LISTEN
AND
LOSE WEIGHT

The Breakthrough Hypnosis
Program for Permanent Weight Loss

GLENN HARROLD

New York   Chicago   San Francisco   Lisbon   London   Madrid   Mexico City
Milan   New Delhi   San Juan   Seoul   Singapore   Sydney   Toronto

Library of Congress Cataloging-in-Publication Data

Harrold, Glenn.
    Listen and lose weight : the breakthrough hypnosis program for permanent
weight loss / Glenn Harrold.
        p.   cm.
    ISBN 978-0-07-149753-4 (alk. paper)
    1. Weight loss.   2. Autogenic training.   I. Title.

RM222.2.H2543   2007
615.8′5122—dc22
                                                                2007026294

1 2 3 4 5 6 7 8 9 10 11 12 13 14 15 16 17 18 19 20 21   FGR/FGR   0 9 8 7

ISBN 978-0-07-149753-4 (book and CD)
MHID   0-07-149753-6 (book and CD)

ISBN 978-0-07-149754-1 (book alone)
MHID   0-07-149754-4 (book alone)

Interior design by Monica Baziuk

McGraw-Hill books are available at special quantity discounts to use as premiums
and sales promotions, or for use in corporate training programs. For more information,
please write to the Director of Special Sales, Professional Publishing, McGraw-Hill, Two
Penn Plaza, New York, NY 10121-2298. Or contact your local bookstore.

The information contained in this book is intended to provide helpful and informative
material on the subject addressed. It is not intended to serve as a replacement for
professional medical advice. Any use of the information in this book is at the reader's
discretion. The author and publisher specifically disclaim any and all liability arising
directly or indirectly from the use or application of any information contained in this
book. A health-care professional should be consulted regarding your specific situation.

This book is printed on acid-free paper.

To everyone who is on the path to improving mind and body. Set yourself free and live the life you deserve.

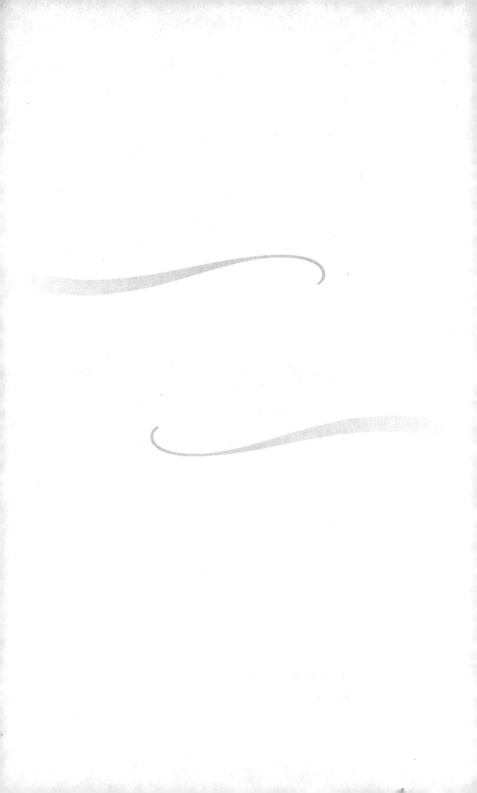

Contents

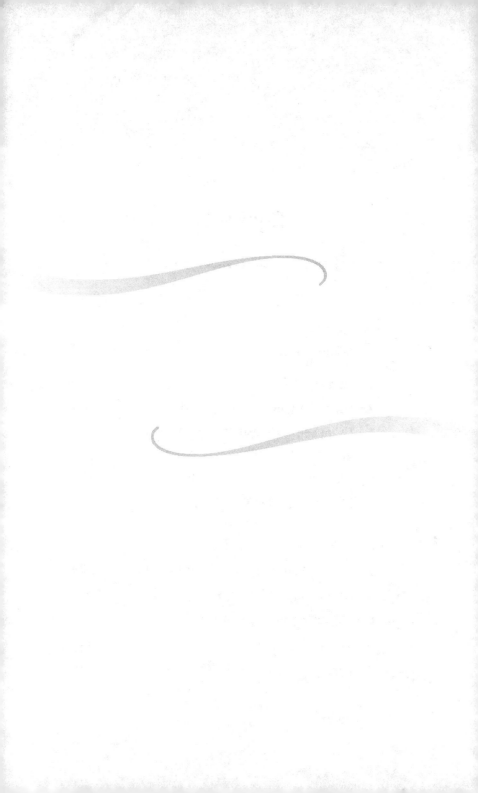

Preface

WELCOME TO *Listen and Lose Weight: The Breakthrough Hypnosis Program for Permanent Weight Loss.* This book and hypnotherapy CD will help you lose weight and maintain a new healthy lifestyle. The fact that you have bought this book means you are determined to reach this goal. Maybe the reason you have not previously succeeded in achieving your weight loss goal is because you did not address the underlying root causes of your weight problems. There is always a root cause driving any bad habit or problem, and being overweight and unfit is simply an accumulation of bad habits. This book and hypnotherapy CD will give you the tools to change those habits forever, providing the catalyst for permanent changes to improve your health and well-being.

Listen and Lose Weight is not a rigid weight loss program or plan that you must adhere to. Rather it covers everything you need to help you create a new, holistic approach to eating and exercise. I'm not a fan of one-size-fits-all programs because in my experience each person's reason for being overweight is unique. My goal with this book is to cover all issues connected with weight control and to help as many people as possible achieve their goals by using psychological reprogramming techniques and motivational guidance.

Learning new skills on both a conscious level and an unconscious level can facilitate changes in behavior very quickly. This is how hypnotherapy works, and you will learn many techniques to help you release negative conditioning and program your mind with positive new beliefs.

When I discovered hypnosis and how effective it can be in changing patterns of behavior, it changed my life. For many years I worked as a musician. In my teens I played bass in a punk band that morphed into a pop band that went on to have an all-too-brief taste of success in the early 1980s. Later on I made a living playing covers in pubs, bars, hotels, and restaurants. One of these gigs was a show in a club where we shared the bill with a stage hypnotist. I had always been fascinated by the power of the mind, and, after watching the show, I decided to learn hypnosis.

However, I didn't want to learn hypnosis just to make people do whacky stuff. I was drawn to hypnosis because of its potential to heal. This is the difference between stage hypnosis and hypnotherapy. The former uses hypnosis largely to entertain while the latter uses hypnosis to help and transform. Once I became qualified in hypnosis,

I went on to build a busy private practice and have gained great personal satisfaction from helping people overcome their problems. I have treated thousands of clients and have dealt with every kind of stress-related problem and all types of phobia. I have helped people lose weight, stop smoking, overcome fears, overcome sleep problems, and build their self-confidence and self-esteem.

After gaining this invaluable grassroots experience, I drew upon my musical background and began making hypnosis CDs, primarily to support my work with my clients. The combination of my hypnotherapy experience and recording knowledge enabled me to make effective CDs, which I sold in many stores. Then I started my own publishing company to market and distribute my materials. I had no marketing or publishing experience but simply used my self-hypnosis skills to help me succeed in business. At the time of writing this book, my hypnosis CDs have sold 500,000 copies worldwide and are one of the world's most downloaded self-help audios.

With *Listen and Lose Weight*, I have used my experience to create a book and CD that contain everything you need to help you lose weight, build self-esteem, and develop a powerful, lasting motivation to take full control of your health and well-being. I wish you all the very best and hope that *Listen and Lose Weight* will be the inspiration you have been seeking.

Best wishes.

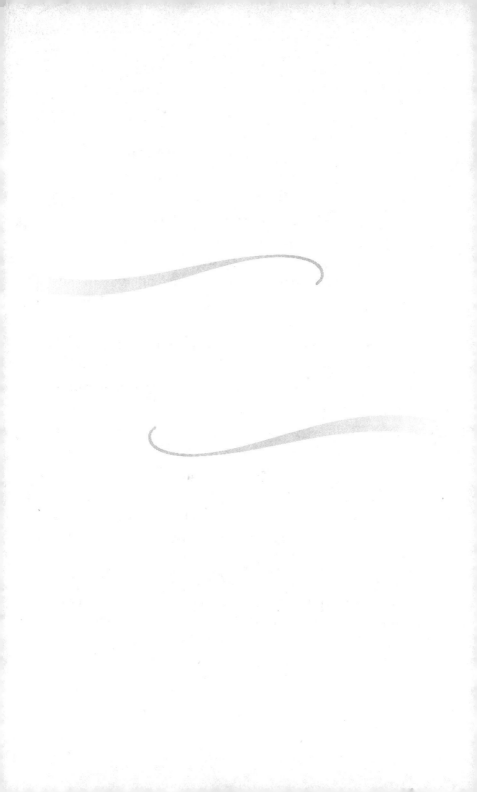

Acknowledgments

———

I WOULD like to thank my editor at McGraw-Hill, Johanna Bowman, for her hard work and attention to detail; Jan Warran-Smith at Diviniti Publishing for her copyedits and guidance; my wife, Aly Harrold, for her advice and for being my sounding board for ideas; and all the staff at Diviniti Publishing for their support.

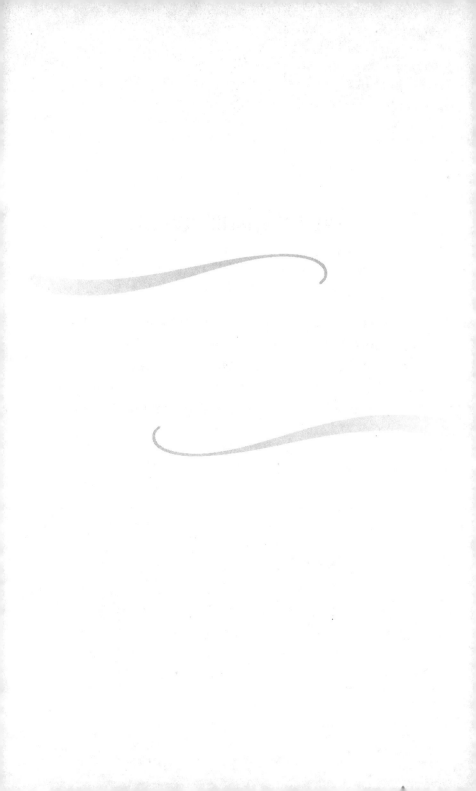

1

How Hypnosis Works

───

There is a misconception that you are out of
control when under hypnosis. The truth is you
are very much in control and in a position to
empower yourself while under hypnosis.

I F YOU read through *Listen and Lose Weight* carefully,
practice the self-hypnosis techniques, and listen regularly to the hypnotherapy CD, you will achieve any
weight loss goal you set for yourself. This will happen
without struggle or conflict. You will simply learn to
reprogram your mind to eat healthily and exercise more.

The two crucial elements to achieving weight loss
are: *Eat smaller amounts of healthy food and exercise regularly.*
Simple, really! How great would it be if this were easy?
Well, it absolutely can be. I want you to know that you

truly deserve to be healthy, happy, and in good shape. This is your right, and you are going to learn to embrace these new beliefs on a deep level. When you do this, you won't need to diet or struggle anymore. Instead, you will automatically accept that you are a healthy eater and in control of your weight. By taking back control in a completely natural way through learning to reprogram your thoughts, you can genuinely learn to love healthy food and exercising, while teaching yourself to dislike sweet, fattening junk food and high-calorie drinks. When you absorb and assimilate these beliefs on a deeper unconscious level, staying in control of your weight becomes natural and easy.

In my hypnotherapy practice the most common problem I help people with is weight loss. Having helped thousands of people achieve their weight loss goals in one-on-one sessions and via my weight loss CDs and DVDs, I have a good understanding of the role the unconscious mind plays in losing weight. Have you ever started on a new weight loss program with great enthusiasm and resolve, only to slip back three months later into those old, destructive eating patterns? The only way to guarantee lasting change is to reprogram your mind. Even the very best weight loss programs only teach you to eat healthily and to exercise on a *conscious* level.

It is said that the conscious part of our brain accounts for about 10 percent of our minds. It seems an awful waste to me that we cart this big brain around but then fail to make full use of it. Well, you are going to learn to tap into the creative, resourceful part of your brain and use more than the standard 10 percent. The key is using the inner worlds of meditation, visualization, and self-hypnosis. This is where your innate power and creativity reside. As you can see, working with a weight loss program on a superficial, conscious level will not create lasting change. To succeed in the long term, you also need to work at a deeper, *unconscious* level.

Losing weight doesn't have to be a struggle anymore. You want to lose weight *and* feel good while you do so. Therefore, enjoying the whole process is important. When you reprogram your thought processes through hypnosis that is exactly what will happen. You will feel good about yourself *and* learn how to develop a powerful new self-esteem and a real motivation to exercise. Having a holistic approach to your health is the key to making a lasting change to your weight.

How Hypnosis and Self-Hypnosis Work

Throughout this book there are a number of self-hypnosis techniques and visualizations designed to help you focus on different weight loss issues.

Don't let the thought of being under hypnosis scare you, as it is often misunderstood. When you experience hypnosis you are simply in an altered state of consciousness. When you go to sleep at night and you drift between consciousness and unconsciousness it feels natural, but as you drift asleep your brain waves are actually slowing. When you go into a hypnotic trance the same thing happens, although you are still aware of your surroundings even as you drift into deeper states. It can sometimes feel as though very little is happening and that you can open your eyes at any time and be wide awake. This is true, but you can still achieve lasting changes even from being in the lightest trance.

Being in an altered state of consciousness or in a hypnotic trance is actually something you will experience naturally many times in your life. For example, just before you fall asleep each night and before you are fully awake in the morning you are in a trance state that everyone on the planet experiences. These morning and evening trance states are called the hypnogogic and hypnopompic states. Daydreaming is another naturally occurring trance state that is familiar to all of us. Now you can learn how to create those states at will to empower yourself and develop a healthy lifestyle.

We all experience hypnosis at least twice a day. The hypnogogic and hypnopompic states are natural trance states that occur as you are waking up and drifting off to sleep every morning and night.

Imagine an iceberg with the tip above the water and the huge bulk below the surface. This is often used to describe the conscious and unconscious minds. We spend most of our time in our conscious thoughts and only sporadically tap into our unconscious mind when we daydream or get creative ideas. The only other time we spend in our unconscious thoughts is when we are sleeping, when our conscious mind has switched off. Learning to connect with your deep unconscious mind by focusing your thoughts can help you in so many different ways to achieve goals, find your creativity, or overcome difficulties.

When you start to use the self-hypnosis and visualization techniques in this book, don't worry if you feel you're not doing it right or not going deep enough into a trance. Affirmations and visualizations are a remarkably effective reprogramming method, and they will still make a big impact on your inner thought processes. Just by closing your eyes, breathing deeply, and really focusing on the affirmations as you say them, you will begin to make significant positive changes in the way you think and feel about your health and well-being.

Don't get concerned about achieving a certain depth of trance. Absorbing suggestion is the crucial element in therapy-based hypnosis, and this can be achieved easily even in very light alpha trance states. The most important part of hypnosis is focusing your attention on a specific goal while you are relaxed and receptive to changes.

Using Hypnosis to Help You Realize Your Goal

Hypnosis can help you achieve your weight loss goal by changing patterns of behavior on a deep level, which

will bring about lasting changes. This will help you create new healthy habits that will become a permanent
part of your life. As I said earlier, working on a weight
loss goal on a purely conscious level will not bring about
lasting changes. Working on a deeper, unconscious level,
however, allows you to create new core beliefs that stay
with you.

When you close your eyes, relax, and practice going
into a deeper trance, you will be drifting into an altered
state of consciousness. So be aware of the occurrence of
this gentle shift in consciousness when you are practicing
self-hypnosis and going into a trance. Hypnosis is often
subtle. It is not the sudden deep trance at the snap of the
fingers that you may have seen performed by stage hyp-
notists. This type of high-profile theatrical induction can
create a misrepresentation. In most normal sessions, the
induction into deeper hypnosis is gradual and controlled
by the person under hypnosis.

How to Use This Book and CD

Don't worry if some of the techniques included here
seem a little unusual to you; with practice you will
soon get the hang of them. You don't need to use every
technique, just use the ones that apply the most to your
situation. However, some techniques such as the future
visualization technique (Chapter 2), the motivation
technique (Chapter 4), and the releasing negative con-

ditioning technique (Chapter 5) are very important and will apply to everyone. Use the techniques in the book that are most relevant to your situation. If your biggest problem is that you eat too much sugary food, then give more attention to the techniques that help you break free of this habit.

The CD that accompanies this book was created specifically to reinforce the book's content. The unique techniques and subtle sound effects have been carefully created for maximum impact. I recommend that you listen to the CD through headphones while lying down so you can absorb all the positive suggestions and affirmations on a deeper level. I also suggest that you start using the CD as soon as possible because the two thirty-minute hypnotherapy sessions on it for weight loss and exercise motivation will give you a great start. Once you feel you are in control, you can use the CD to reinforce your goals whenever you feel the need.

Track 1, "Lose Weight Now," will help you release negative conditioning, build your self-esteem, create a powerful future visualization, and develop healthy eating patterns. Track 2, "Feel Motivated to Exercise," will help you become much more active and build a powerful desire to exercise regularly. When you have a deep-rooted belief that you *love* exercising, losing weight and maintaining fitness becomes effortless. If you want to focus more on weight loss, healthy eating, and self-esteem, listen regularly to Track 1 on the CD. If you want to focus on building a strong exercise motivation, use Track 2 more often. If you want to focus equally on both areas, you may want to alternate tracks each day. (For more guidelines on how to use the CD, see Appendix A.)

The background sound effects on each hypnotherapy track have been created in certain keys and frequencies, and they help to guide you into a deep state of mental and physical relaxation. In this very receptive and relaxed state, you will be given a number of posthypnotic and direct suggestions to help you free yourself from poor conditioning, build your self-esteem, and lose weight.

Toward the end of both tracks, you will be instructed to repeat special hypnotic affirmations to help you create a new healthy lifestyle. When you repeat these affirmations, say them with conviction and believe they are a reality. The stronger the feelings you create, the more effective the affirmations will be. So really put your heart and soul into embracing these positive new beliefs.

The stronger the feelings you create, the more effective the affirmations will be. So really put your heart and soul into embracing these positive new beliefs.

In addition to using your feelings and emotions, the other key to absorbing hypnotic suggestion is "compounding." This means that the more you hear the suggestions on the CD as well as use the self-hypnosis techniques in this book, the quicker your unconscious mind will get the message. You will then respond to the suggestions automatically in your everyday life.

There are also a number of echoed background affirmations on both CD tracks, which pan from left to right in your headphones. This deeply relaxing and powerful method of delivering multiple suggestions simultaneously to the unconscious mind can facilitate positive changes very quickly. At the end of each recording, you will be gently brought back to full waking consciousness with a combination of suggestion and music. There are also a number of positive subliminal suggestions, which are embedded in the fade-out music and facilitate the overall effect. These subliminal suggestions are the same as the affirmation phrases on pages 150 and 151 of Appendix B.

There are no hard and fast rules as to how long the CD should be used. The hypnosis CD works differently for each individual. It is impossible to give an estimate for the number of times you should use it, but after listening a few times you should begin to notice some positive changes. The positive changes may be instant and dramatic or a gradual, subtle progression into new patterns of behavior. For maximum effect, listen to the CD on a daily basis until you feel you have achieved your goals—in this case, eating healthily and exercising regularly. You can also continue listening even after you reach your goals because doing so helps reinforce what you have learned.

If you fall asleep listening to the CD but still hear the count to ten at the end of the track, you have probably been in a deep trance throughout. In this state you will still absorb all the suggestions on an unconscious level. If you don't hear the count at the end, you have probably drifted into a deep sleep at some point. In this case, you will absorb the suggestions only to the point where you went into a deeper sleep. If this happens, avoid listening when you are tired.

Your Power of Choice

There are many reasons why people develop poor eating habits, but it is important to remember that you have power of choice. You can choose right now to make changes to the way you eat and exercise. Whatever has happened in the past, you no longer need to let that poor conditioning or bad experience control your life. There are a number of techniques in this book and on the CD to help you overcome negative conditioning. It doesn't make sense to allow events from your past to mess up your life now. You can go forward from here with a clean slate *and* learn to believe that you deserve to be fit, healthy, and in good shape.

Say that to yourself now: "I deserve to be fit, healthy, and in good shape." If it feels good when you say it now, then that's fine. If at this point affirming this phrase feels uncomfortable, don't worry—after reading this book and using the CD, you will be saying and believing it *and* feeling very good as you do so.

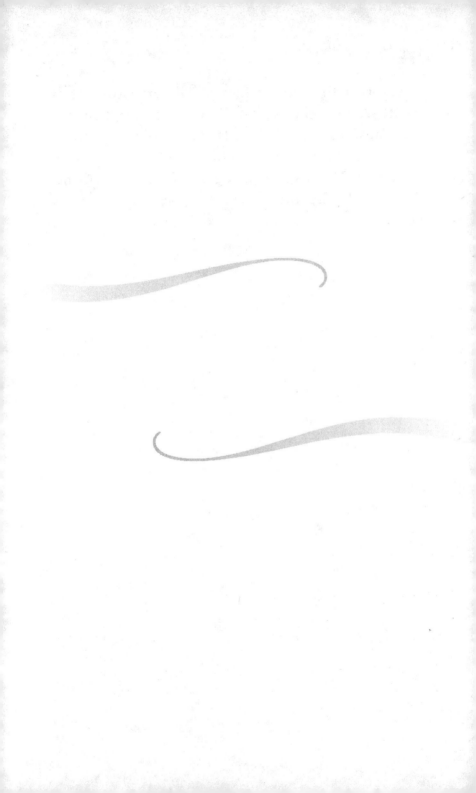

2

Supercharging Your Weight Loss Goal

Visualizing your weight loss goal and creating a clear image in your mind of how you will look and feel when you reach your goal is very important.

HYPNOTHERAPY CAN help anyone achieve permanent results. The only people who can't be helped are those who don't want help. Sometimes people refuse help, preferring to wallow in their own self-pity and neglect, which is usually a result of negative conditioning in their past. But, if you have the desire, you can overcome any bad conditioning. It comes down to how much you want it, and you have to be truthful. If someone is overweight and doesn't want to change, then there is little anyone can do to help. The desire to change has to come from within. If you have that spark of desire, then anything is possible.

You are going to learn to build a powerful and lasting inner desire to lose weight and become fit and healthy. You are not going to discuss it with anyone or try to impress others when you lose a few pounds here and there. This journey is for you and you alone. You are going to learn to remain disciplined and focused.

> "To lengthen thy Life, lessen thy meals."
> —Benjamin Franklin

Write down the three main reasons why you are now choosing to lose weight and become fit. Perhaps you want to lose weight for your health or because you want to be more active with your children. If it helps, close your eyes and think about your priorities and why it is important for you to lose weight and become fit.

_____

_____

_____

Now write down the three main things you would really love to change, for example, to have more energy, to have a better body shape, or to feel more attractive. Whatever they are, write down the most important things that apply to you.

_____

_____

_____

Now that you have clarified your reasons for choosing to lose weight and the things you aim to change, you can move forward with these in mind. When you genuinely have the desire to lose weight, you can begin to create new healthy routines and incorporate into your daily life many of the techniques that you will learn in this book. This can be very enjoyable because you will be empowering yourself on a deep level, which can also have a positive impact in so many other areas of your life.

> *You are going to learn to build a powerful and lasting inner desire to lose weight and become fit and healthy.*

Defining Your Goal

Next you need to determine your weight loss goal. What is your ideal healthy weight? Think carefully about your ideal target weight and don't put a limit on your goal. Even if you weigh 300 pounds, it is possible for you to reach a weight of 170 pounds. Take a moment now to decide on your ideal target weight.

Once you have a clear weight goal in mind, focus on a future date by which you will reach your target weight. Be realistic at this point, because losing weight too quickly can be counterproductive. Most diets fail because of one simple fact: your mind takes time to adjust to a new self-image. So if you lose a lot of weight too quickly, your mind may not adjust to your physical changes at the same speed. It may not recognize your new image because it hasn't caught up. This can create conflict and have a detrimental effect, which in the long term can result in weight fluctuations and a failure to reach and maintain a healthy weight.

> "To climb steep hills requires a slow pace at first."
> —William Shakespeare

Always remember that for a lasting result, the best and most natural way to lose weight is slowly and steadily.

If you are 170 pounds now and your target weight is 140 pounds, allow yourself a comfortable six months to achieve this target. If you have a greater target—for example, to go from 250 pounds to 150 pounds—then allow eighteen to twenty-four months to achieve this because you are looking to shed about a third of your body weight and will need to do so carefully. The message is not to rush; think of this as a holistic journey in which you are empowering your mind and body more and more every day.

> *The best and most natural way to lose weight is slowly and steadily.*

When you have decided upon your ideal target weight and time frame, write it down. This is a key step, so please don't overlook it. Spend a few minutes now on setting a realistic goal. Write: On [future date], I will weigh [your ideal target weight]:

On _____ , I will weigh _____ .

Write your goal on several pieces of paper and put them where you will read them each day. Good places are next to your bed or bathroom mirror, for instance, because you need to see your goal regularly. You can even add your goal to your mobile phone or post it in your workspace or car. The more you see and read your goal, the better. The key to hypnosis and reprogramming your mind is compounding new beliefs through repetition. Seeing your future date and weight goal every day in print is important, because it compounds your determination and desire to achieve your goal every time you read it. Again, it is crucial to stay focused on your goals.

All of these small steps are going to add up to a powerful, lasting solution, which will give you total control of your weight like never before. It will completely take the struggle out of the equation. After using the CD and self-hypnosis techniques, your habits will start to change. You may find yourself automatically turning down the offer of cake or chocolate, or you may feel an inner pull driving you to take up a healthy activity. When you add all of the small steps and techniques together, I guarantee things will change easily and effortlessly. When you create a program that confirms you are a fit and healthy person, this is exactly what you will become.

Using Your Creative Mind

Using visual imagery is a very powerful way of absorbing beliefs into your unconscious mind. Regular visualization will help you remain focused and change your mind's perception of your self-image, which will make changing habits easier. Be creative and make your visualizations colorful and elaborate, with as much detail as possible. Immerse yourself *totally* in the visualizations; use all of your senses to make them realistic and, most important, put your feelings strongly into it. When you see yourself at your target weight looking and feeling great, go into detail and see all the things that have changed for the better now you are at this new weight.

VISUALIZATION TIP

You can use visualization techniques to prepare yourself for future events, such as an exam, a sporting event, public speaking, or business and social occasions. I always feel for people when they blow a big opportunity through nerves or anxiety. Learning these techniques can help absolutely anyone overcome anxiety in pressure situations.

When you visualize a future event you can even run the images in your mind like a short film using as much detail as possible. For instance, if you are going to a wedding in six months, see yourself looking fantastic in a great new outfit. Envision yourself at the wedding having a wonderful, happy time. Feel your clothes against your skin, and notice how good you look and feel. Make the whole picture bright and clear, and use as many of your senses as you can—the more vividly you use your imagination the better. Most important, always see yourself in a completely positive light—looking good, feeling in control, and expressing yourself clearly and confidently.

Visualizing Your Goal

Your next building block is to *visualize* yourself at your future target weight. A key ingredient in mind programming is that the human mind doesn't distinguish between what is real and what is imagined, so when you create a visualization, your mind will accept it as a reality. Studies have actually proven that even by visualizing exercise workouts, your body will respond and show signs of increased conditioning and muscle toning. A scientific study at the Cleveland Clinic Foundation in Ohio found that volunteers who took part in mental workouts five times a week where they visualized lifting weights actually increased their biceps by 13.5 percent on average. And, their gains lasted for three months after they stopped the mental exercise regime.

> "Imagination is
> more important
> than knowledge."
> —Albert Einstein

By using the creative power of your imagination and visualizing yourself at your target weight shape and size, your unconscious mind will believe that this is a reality now. When your mind adjusts to a new body image in this way, you will then take unconscious steps to create the physical reality. This is why losing weight by using self-hypnosis and visualization is so easy—it takes the struggle out of the process.

The following technique is a good starting point in learning to program yourself with positive thoughts and to familiarize yourself with going into a gentle trance. Self-hypnosis is a very powerful state of mind and something anyone can use at any time. While you will be reprogramming your mind when you use the CD, you can also build the future visualization technique into your daily routines.

You will learn more about hypnosis throughout the book. Once you are more experienced in the ways of self-hypnosis, you can revisit this script and develop this technique, which is about creating a strong intention so that your mind has a clear image of your ideal weight shape and size.

Stop at this point and read the future visualization technique script through a few times until you know what to do. Then practice this visualization every day—ideally for twenty-one days. Then you can refresh it every now and again. As with all things, practice makes perfect, and you will find that the more you practice the deeper you will go and the better you will get at making the visualization real. You can spend as little as ten minutes creating the images and feelings, or you can spend longer if you prefer. The key is repeating the visualization each day so that you strengthen your new mental program.

You may find creative ideas will come to you once you have begun to practice the future visualization technique. It may be that you get new ideas to exercise more a day or two after you try future visualization. Practice this technique often, especially at the beginning of your journey. You will find that your images and feelings become more positive each time you do so.

Future Visualization Technique

GO TO A quiet darkened room where there are no distractions. Take a moment to get in a comfortable position, close your eyes, and focus your attention on your breathing. Begin breathing slowly and deeply in through your nose and out through your mouth in a circular breathing motion. Breathe away any tension left in your body with every slow breath out and allow yourself to relax more and more.

Continue this breathing pattern a dozen or more times and clear away any unwanted thoughts so that your mind becomes still and quiet. Simply focus on the stillness of the moment.

With your mind still and quiet, imagine going forward in time, into your future to the date that you have set to reach your target weight. Stay deeply relaxed and focus on this point in time.

As you go forward into the future, visualize yourself at your target weight looking slimmer, fitter, and healthier. Amplify the positive feelings and make the image big, bright, and clear.

See yourself at this new weight standing in front of a full-length mirror dressed in a brand-new outfit. You look so good and feel so attractive and confident at this new shape and size. Use all of your senses to make it real. Feel the clothes brush against your skin; notice the pleasant aroma of the new clothing. Run your hands down your slim physique and praise yourself as you do so.

Now accept on every level that this is what you deserve. Hold this picture in your mind and affirm to yourself silently or out loud:

- ➤ I love being fit and healthy.
- ➤ I love being in control of my weight.

Accept that you have lost any need or desire for sickly sweet, fattening food and that you love looking so attractive and feeling so healthy at this new weight. Take a moment now just to really enjoy this positive feeling.

When you do this, these feelings and images will sink into your unconscious mind and become a part of your inner reality.

Your unconscious mind will see this positive image of yourself at your ideal weight and accept it as real, which will help you work toward your goal with ease.

When you are ready to finish, allow your mind to clear by slowly counting up to ten, open your eyes, and come back to full waking consciousness. When you reach ten, every part of you will be back in the here and now.

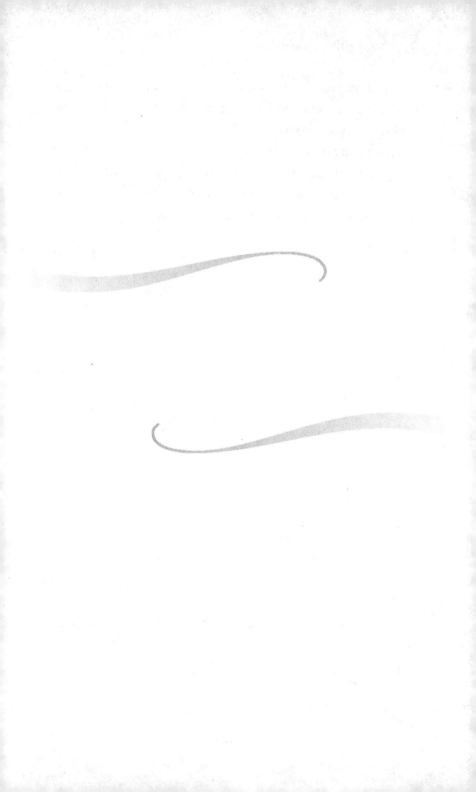

3

Using Self-Hypnosis and Affirmations for Lasting Results

Feel the affirmations as you repeat them—draw them inside you and let every cell in your mind and body resonate with positive feeling and emotion.

T HE KEY to your success is in reprogramming your old thought patterns. If you can exercise regularly and eat healthily, you will lose weight. It is as simple as that. Now imagine if this were easy to do, as though it were second nature to you. Imagine you had no desire for sweets, chocolate, French fries, soft drinks, or any other fattening foods. These are foods your body doesn't need or want, and you can easily live a perfectly happy life without ever thinking about them again. This is an easy mind-set to create, and I will show you how in this chapter.

Do you remember the first time you learned to do something new, for example, drive a new car? You may have driven for years, but learning all about a new, unfamiliar car can be frustrating. How do you turn on the lights or the windshield wipers? Is the gas tank filled from the left or right side? Programming the clock and radio the first time can take a while. The first trip or two can be difficult. But then you learn where everything is and how it all works, and the mechanics become almost an automatic, unconscious process.

You can use that same inherent learning ability to teach yourself to love exercising and healthy food. You can learn to love feeling fit and healthy and to find fattening food repulsive. Whatever your weight loss aims, you can reprogram your mind in specific ways to help you to achieve your goals. Learning these new habits is a matter of repetition.

> "It is health that is real wealth and not pieces of gold and silver."
> —Mahatma Gandhi

The more you visualize and absorb these affirmations, the quicker you create the new inner belief. It is also very enjoyable because you will be creating very relaxing mental states that benefit your general health and well-being.

How Affirmations Work

A goal is a specific target that you set for yourself to achieve within a fixed time frame. An affirmation is a statement of intent that you repeat to yourself over and over again. Affirmations should be words and phrases that are stated in a clear and concise way with a positive emphasis. Whenever you use your affirmations, feel as though you are drawing the words inside you, as though you are teaching the inner part of yourself a new belief. You must always state affirmations in the present tense and focus on them as if they are a reality now.

The wording of your affirmations must be decided upon before you begin a self-hypnosis session, and you must work on only one goal at a time. For example, don't work on releasing a fear and losing weight in the same session. While you can use a number of affirmations in one session, they must all relate to the one chosen goal for that session.

When deciding beforehand on your affirmations, always state them *as if they are a reality and in the present*. This is very important because your unconscious mind will believe *exactly* what it is told. For example:

Do *not* say: "I want to be fit and healthy."
Do say: "I *love* being fit and healthy." Or, "I *am* fit and healthy."

You could use the word *feeling* if your preferred sense is kinesthetic (feeling). For example:

Do say: "I *love feeling* fit and healthy."

You must make affirmations completely unambiguous and always accentuate the positive. I tend to use the words "I love to . . ." to begin many of my affirmations because *love* is a powerful, emotive word, and I find this type of affirmation has a profound impact.

> *You must make affirmations completely unambiguous and always accentuate the positive.*

To make them stronger, really *feel* the affirmations as you repeat them. Draw them inside you and let every cell in your mind and body resonate with positive feelings and emotion. Imagine every part of you is repeating the affirmations with complete conviction and total belief in what you are stating. Even if this feels a bit odd at first, stay with it. Remember, your unconscious mind believes exactly what it is told. You are creating new positive beliefs that will be accepted exactly as they are, without any analysis, by your unconscious mind. That is why it is very important to take time and care to word your affirmations correctly.

Writing down your goals and affirmations is very important because it gives the words power and meaning, reminding you constantly of where you are heading. It also spells out your intent loud and clear, adding clarity to your aims and helping to compound your new belief structures.

Using Self-Hypnosis to Supercharge Your Affirmations

Make a mental note of two or three short affirmations before you begin self-hypnosis. For example:

- I am in full control of my weight.
- I deserve to be fit and healthy.
- I love to exercise regularly and keep fit.

Find a quiet room where you will not be disturbed, and make yourself as comfortable as possible. Once you get skilled at self-hypnosis, you can use it in busy places where there are noises and distractions. With practice you will find it easy to block out distractions and be able to focus your mind intently.

Tell yourself silently or out loud that you are going to practice self-hypnosis and state how long you want to remain in the trance. Fifteen to twenty minutes is fine to begin with. However, after a little practice you may decide to make your sessions last longer.

Close your eyes and begin to breathe very slowly and deeply—in through your nose and out through your mouth. At the top of your breath, hold it for three seconds and then count to five on every breath out. As you breathe out, imagine you are breathing away any nervous tension left in your body.

Breathe from your diaphragm (lower chest area) and not from the upper chest. Watch what happens to your body as you breathe. If you are breathing properly, your stomach will go out as you breathe in and go in as you breathe out. This can take a little practice if you are unused to diaphragmatic breathing. Continue this breathing pattern ten or more times, or as long as it takes for you to feel completely relaxed.

Allow your mind to go completely blank. Don't worry if you still get any unwanted thoughts in your mind; tell yourself not to fight them because they will soon drift away again.

Deepening the Trance State

By now you will already be in a light trance state. A good technique to guide yourself deeper into a trance is to count down silently and mentally from ten to one. Feel every muscle in your body relax more and more with each descending number. Leave about five seconds between each number, or count each number down on every second or third breath out. To enhance this you can also use visualization techniques. For example, imagine you are traveling down ten flights in an escalator or stepping down ten steps into a beautiful garden. Use whatever feels right for you. Count down with each flight or step, going deeper into the trance with each number.

Affirming Your Goal

When you feel mentally and physically relaxed, slowly repeat your affirmations over and over in your mind, using your feelings to give them real strength. Create a rhythm with your breathing, saying the affirmation on each breath out like a chant or mantra. As you repeat your affirmations, you can also bring in the images of yourself at your ideal weight. Even though you may not be at your ideal weight right now, when you affirm and visualize it is important that you see yourself clearly at your ideal weight, shape, and size. Take plenty of time to do this.

Bringing Yourself Back to Full Consciousness

When you feel it is time to wake up, all you need to do is slowly and mentally count up from one to ten. Tell yourself you are becoming more awake with each number. When you reach ten, your eyes will open and you will be wide awake with a feeling of total well-being.

If you practice this process before going to sleep, you do not need to count up from one to ten. Simply tell yourself before you begin your session that the trance will turn into a deep, natural sleep from which you will wake in the morning feeling positive and refreshed.

Think of the analogy of reprogramming a computer with new data. What you put into it is going to come

SELF-HYPNOSIS TIP

When you first practice self-hypnosis, do not worry if you don't think that much has happened, that you didn't feel any different, or that you could not see much in the visualization. You will be surprised at how effective a suggestion can be in even the lightest of trances. The power of the unconscious mind works in a very subtle way. Just the fact that you went somewhere quiet and centered yourself by closing your eyes and relaxing will have benefited you.

The most important thing to remember is to enjoy the process and to have faith, because as with all things, the more you practice the better you become!

back out. Totally immerse yourself in your aims. When you are in a trance, use all of your senses to compound the phrases and make your affirmations and visualizations colorful and real. Do not worry if you are not good at visualizing; you may have a different dominant sense. Most people are visual, but others absorb information more easily through another sense—feeling, hearing, smell, or even taste. That is why it is important to use all

of your senses when visualizing so that your more dominant sense will help you to absorb the new beliefs at a
deeper level.

Hypnotherapy Case Study

One thing I realized early on is that the power of hypnosis
is not about the hypnotherapist. It is about the belief of
the individual and how much he or she wants his or her
goal to happen. One of my first clients demonstrated this
perfectly.

This gentleman was very nervous about being hypnotized but was desperate to stop smoking for health reasons.
We discussed all the common myths about hypnosis, and
I reassured him that the experience would be nothing like
the hypnosis stage shows he'd seen. I explained he would be
in control at all times and that I was simply guiding him.

We were soon getting on fine, and his nerves were
disappearing. We even began discussing his hobbies and
were in the middle of talking about football, when all of
a sudden he sat bolt upright in his chair and fixed his eyes
on mine. He then began swaying from side to side and
said slowly, "Oh, you're doing it to me now!" He continued to sway with his eyes locked on mine, believing
that I had already started to hypnotize him. He had gone
into the deepest trance I'd ever witnessed, but because I
hadn't even begun the induction stage of my hypnotherapy session I knew it was nothing that I had done. Being

a relatively inexperienced hypnotherapist at that time, I was initially bewildered. This spontaneous deep trance phenomenon had not been covered in my training!

I instructed him to lie down on the couch, which he duly did. I then spent the next thirty minutes going through my induction script, which I later realized was completely unnecessary. He was already in a very receptive state and would have accepted suggestions easily at that point. I eventually guided him out of the trance, and he said he felt great and happily went on his way. He was relieved, and I was confused! This gentleman had in effect put himself into a trance state because he believed I had started to induct him.

Unusual as it was, the session was a success, as I later heard from a family member that he remained a non-smoker since that day. It made me realize that the real power in hypnosis lies with the individual, about his or her perception of hypnosis and about what that individual believes he or she can achieve. Belief is everything. Create the belief first, and the reality will follow.

The Power of Your Mind

Never underestimate the power you have inside you. Your mind has truly incredible potential. All around the world there are stories of humans achieving feats that are seemingly impossible. There are documented cases of mothers being able to summon superhuman strength to lift a car off the ground to save their children trapped underneath. When the mother sees her child in danger she doesn't stop and think, *I can't lift that car because it weighs too much*. The only thought in her mind is to save her child; the fact that the car is too heavy to lift never enters her thinking. This is the key to how she can do it—there is not a doubt in her mind and she is totally focused on lifting the car. Through extreme focus and sheer force of will, the mother is able to summon the strength to lift a car weighing more than a ton.

The survival instinct is the most powerful driver humans possess, and when this is threatened, in extreme circumstances, we can do things that defy logic. When we are in serious danger, our focus becomes heightened and we enter an altered state of consciousness. In this altered state we can utilize incredible strength and power. By using self-hypnosis you will be able to engage your mind in a similar way and achieve so much. Think of the story of the mother lifting the car as a metaphor for your journey to health and fitness. Never put a limit on what you can do. You can achieve absolutely anything when you learn to focus your mind.

> *Never underestimate the power you have inside you. Your mind has truly incredible potential.*

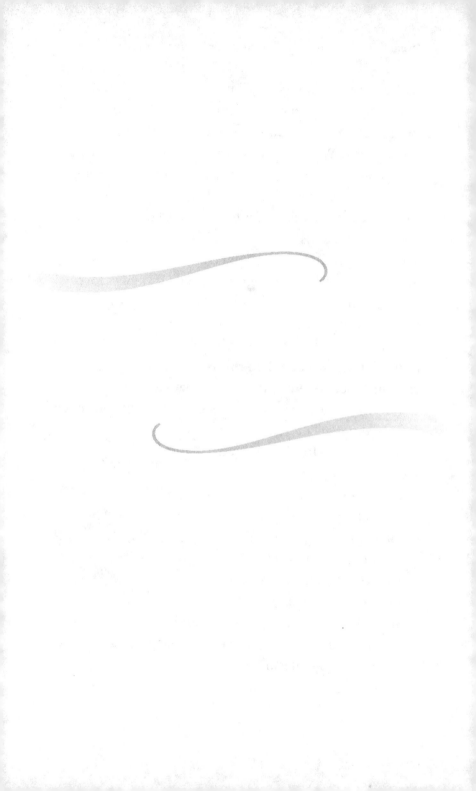

4

Discovering Your
True Motivation

—

Avoid discussing your weight loss aims. If any-

one asks you about weight loss, just say

you are creating a healthier lifestyle.

O NE THING to be clear about is that for most people, being overweight is a choice. It is not an affliction or an illness; it is merely an accumulation of bad habits. There are exceptions to this, of course, but for the major-ity of overweight people, it has become a lifestyle choice.

If you are overweight, you have to take personal responsibility and make changes inside. You give your power away by asking others to change things for you rather than admitting to yourself, *Okay, I've created this problem so I am going to put it right.* Be true to yourself, and put all your energy into making positive personal changes that improve the quality of your life. By creating a healthy holistic lifestyle, you can make changes and be the person you are supposed to be. It simply means consistently making the right choices for the good of your health.

Harnessing Your Energy

It is also very important not to discuss your weight loss goals with other people. It is okay to tell them how you did it *after* your have achieved your weight goal, but in the early stages say little or nothing. Idle chatter dissipates the energy you are going to build as you progress. While friends and family can be well meaning, they can also hold you back because people are not always comfortable when their nearest and dearest make changes, even positive ones!

> "Always aim at complete harmony of thought and word and deed."
> —*Mahatma Gandhi*

This is going to be a solo journey, something that first and foremost you are doing for yourself. Doing anything alone can be difficult at times because when you make a shift like this, you can sometimes distance yourself from people close to you. When you start to make personal changes—even though they are positive ones—you may find some relationships change and this can be tough and testing. It is because people around you can feel insecure when you change, as they may fear losing you. In some cases it can highlight their own failings and lack of motivation.

You have to move on regardless because being fit and healthy is more important than trying to keep others happy. So avoid getting held back because of other people's insecurities. Those who really care about you will always come around if they see you changing for the right reasons, and you will win their respect in the end. You need to continue on your journey without debate or discussion, in a silent and disciplined way. It matters not what others think provided you are improving your quality of life in a positive way.

The following metaphor sums up this weird quirk of human behavior: A man goes into a restaurant where he notices a large bucket full of live crabs. He notices that one crab is climbing up the bucket wall, and it looks like he is going to escape. So the man informs the waiter. The waiter tells the man that the crab will never escape because every time one gets near the top, the other crabs in the bucket will always pull it back.

> *While you may encounter some resistance and negativity on your journey, you will also secretly inspire others and many will be very proud of you.*

The moral to this story—and one to remember—is never to allow others to hold you back. You are going to achieve your target weight and become happier and more fulfilled regardless of what anyone else says or thinks. Even though you may encounter some resistance and negativity on your journey, you will also secretly inspire people and many will be very proud of you. The following short self-protection technique can help you feel protected from any negative outside energy. You can use it to deflect criticism or if others try to hold you back.

Self-Protection Technique

CLOSE YOUR EYES and take a few slow deep breaths. Now imagine you are surrounded by a white protective light. Visualize a protective energy field all around your body, as though you have stepped inside a white bubble of pure healing light. When you imagine this light around you, you will feel completely safe and secure. No negative energy can pass through this protective shield. If anyone criticizes you or tries to knock you down, it will bounce off your protective shield and have no effect on you. Only positive thoughts and energy can pass through your protective light.

Anytime you imagine you are inside this white bubble in your everyday life, you will immediately feel safe and secure and protected from outside negativity or from people who are an energy drain.

This self-protection technique is another little building block should you need it. It may seem very simple, but never underestimate the power of simple visualizations. When you visualize and focus, you are tapping into that powerful creative part of your mind that knows no limitation.

The following case study demonstrates how powerful a simple technique like this can be. A few years ago a lady booked a session of hypnotherapy with me at one of my clinics. Her problem was rather unusual in that it involved her ex-boyfriend. This man had found it hard to accept that their relationship was over and had begun stalking her. This naturally terrified her, and after one particularly frightening incident, she had a court issue a restraining order against him. However, he ignored this and continued to terrify her.

When she first came to my clinic, one of the techniques we worked on was the white light self-protection technique. This worked well, and so I developed the technique each time I hypnotized her and gave her many posthypnotic suggestions, telling her that she would now feel safe and secure and have a powerful protective energy around her.

After three or four sessions, she felt much stronger in herself and said that the fear she had for this man was not there anymore. She was still wary but no longer felt terrorized twenty-four hours a day. I felt that under the circumstances the sessions had been successful because she was much more in control of her thoughts and feelings.

A few months passed. Then one day she called to say an amazing thing had happened. A few days previously, her ex and another man had confronted her in the street. He stood a few yards in front of her with a knife in his hand and began making threats. She said at this point she became very frightened but refused to give in to him or show any fear. Instead she immediately began to imagine and feel the white light surrounding and protecting her.

Something inexplicable happened at this point. She said the two men stopped in their tracks, and one turned to the other and said, "Look at that white light around her." They then turned around and took off. She never saw or heard from this man again. She was amazed and delighted.

I can't explain what happened, nor would I try to. All I can say is that the story was relayed to me first-hand by this client, a well-educated schoolteacher and, in my opinion, not the type to invent such things. She had been visualizing the protective white light for a number of weeks before this incident took place. She also had gained a lot of strength and self-empowerment from the hypnotherapy sessions. Whether or not her stalker saw the light doesn't really matter. Through her inner work, she had become empowered again and was giving off a completely different energy.

Through hypnotherapy I have seen minor miracles like this that are hard to explain. You can never put a limitation on the potential we all have inside of us. I believe we all have infinite talents and unique creative gifts. This unlimited creativity can be accessed when we quiet the chatter of our conscious mind and go deep inside to the powerful, resourceful part of ourselves.

No More Excuses

You aren't going to make lasting changes if you are kidding yourself or your friends or family about your weight loss goals. You need to become genuinely determined to overcome any unhealthy eating patterns and reach your ideal weight. This is not about impressing or pleasing others; you are doing this for yourself. You simply decide to lose weight and achieve your target or you don't. It comes down to the power of choice and being honest about your aims. Think

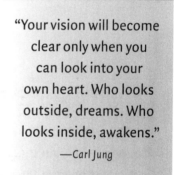

"Your vision will become clear only when you can look into your own heart. Who looks outside, dreams. Who looks inside, awakens."
—Carl Jung

how fortunate you are to have the freedom of choice. You can make a simple decision now that will empower you in so many ways.

Be truthful with yourself now, and make the decision from the bottom of your heart. It is no good saying, "Yes, I am going to do this," but still having loads of treats in your kitchen just waiting to be devoured the next time you think you have done something good! By now you should be well on the way to eliminating these old hab-

> "An invincible determi-
> nation can accomplish
> almost anything and in
> this lies the great dis-
> tinction between great
> men and little men."
>
> —Thomas Fuller

its. Food is not about treating yourself. You must create the mind-set whereby you eat to live, not live to eat.

I know someone who is always telling people that he is eating healthily and exercising yet he complains that he can never lose weight. Everyone around him knows he overin-

dulges and doesn't really exercise, but he continues to

Weight Loss Technique

CLOSE YOUR EYES now and take a few slow deep breaths. Connect with your inner self and the truthful part of you. This is the part of you that knows what is best for you and has real integrity. Then affirm to yourself:

- I love being in control of my eating habits.
- I love being fit and healthy.

Repeat these sentences over and over with real feeling so that every cell in your body resonates with this truth.

peddle his hard luck story. You have to be honest with yourself. If you eat healthy, nonfattening food in small amounts and exercise regularly, you will lose weight. It is as simple as that. So avoid complicating this simple truth.

I mentioned briefly that you must avoid discussing your weight loss aims, and I will emphasize this point again. If anyone asks you about weight loss, just say you are creating a healthier lifestyle. Do not talk about your weight and definitely do not say you are dieting. If anyone asks if you are on a diet, respond with a polite no. If they ask you directly if you have lost weight, say that you think you may have. Then change the subject and forget about it.

In this day and age people can be obsessive about the weights of others. How often do we see magazines and newspapers focusing on a celebrity who has lost lots of weight? Then a year later when the same celebrity has ballooned in weight, these same publications give him or her a hard time and publicly humiliate that person. Journal-

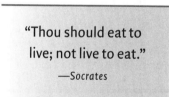

"Thou should eat to live; not live to eat."
—*Socrates*

ists argue that it is what people want to read. Maybe it is—who knows? It does, however, highlight the need for you to play things down and keep quiet about your weight goals. On your journey avoid making bold statements about your weight loss or trying to impress. Yours is a disciplined, silent quest for self-empowerment.

Clarifying Your Motivation

We all have the potential to make changes and succeed in our lives. To succeed at any goal means becoming single-minded and focused. Once again I want you to focus on the area of motivation and really think about why you want to reach your target weight now. What are the reasons for making this permanent change in your life? Maybe it is for health reasons, or because you want to look and feel good about your appearance. Ask yourself now: What is it that is motivating me? Why do I want to achieve my goal? How badly do I want to achieve my goal? What is going to keep me motivated if times get tough?

> *Yours is a disciplined, silent quest for self-empowerment.*

Sometimes your motivation can come from wanting to look good at an upcoming holiday, wedding, or party. It is fine to focus on things like this to galvanize you in the short term, but remember that your long-term aim must always be to create a permanent, holistic healthy lifestyle.

Write down now all the reasons why you want to reach your target weight. Go into detail and list as many motivators as possible.

Hopefully, you have used a few of the techniques in this book and have listened to the CD a few times by now, and you should be developing some useful therapy skills. Use the following motivation technique to create a clear decision now to reach and maintain your target weight. This technique will help focus your mind and build an unstoppable determination to lose weight and achieve your goal. Remember, when you create the thought, the feelings follow and the actual reality will happen later. You always start with the thought, then the deed, and then the goal will follow. Read the technique through a few times before you practice it.

It is important to use this technique regularly so your determination grows and creates a momentum that becomes unstoppable. You are going to build a powerful, lasting inner desire to lose weight and become fit and healthy. You are not going to try to impress others when you lose a few pounds here and there. This is a silent, disciplined journey where you learn to take back control and live the healthy life that you fully deserve.

This holistic weight loss approach will improve the quality of your life, so you must be totally honest with yourself and clear in your aims.

Motivation Technique

CLOSE YOUR EYES and take a few very slow, deep breaths, relaxing your mind and body. Breathe away any stress and relax with each breath out. Now think of a time in your life when you were very determined, a time when you had a fire in your belly because you wanted to achieve a goal. Maybe you wanted something so badly that it almost hurt. It must have been a positive goal with a positive outcome. Take a moment to think of such a time now.

Remember that time and connect with all those feelings of determination you had and the strong desire to succeed. Remember how you felt, what you saw, the things you heard. Bring these feelings back with you now, and remember clearly how it feels to be so completely single-minded and set on a goal. Feel that determination again right now resonating through every cell in your mind and body.

Now focus all of these feelings on your goal of reaching your desired target weight. Affirm to yourself that you are making a clear choice now to achieve your weight loss goal.

At this point repeat the following affirmations to yourself silently or out loud. Remember to use your feelings to make the affirmations even stronger and repeat them in sequence in a slow, steady rhythm.

- ➤ I have a powerful desire to reach my weight loss goal.
- ➤ My motivation to become fit and healthy grows stronger every day.
- ➤ I love to succeed.

Now relax your mind and bring back the picture of your-self dressed in your ideal outfit. As you do so, the feelings and images will sink deeply into your unconscious mind and become a part of your inner reality. When you are ready to awaken, slowly count from one to ten, open your eyes, and come back to full waking consciousness.

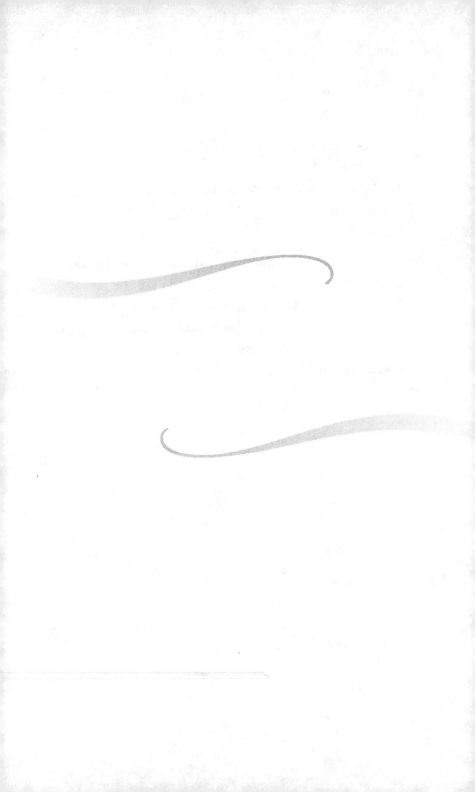

5

Freeing Yourself from Negative Conditioning

Reprogramming your thoughts is an enjoyable

process. You do not have to think about food; rather,

you are focusing your mind on specific aims.

O NE OF the biggest hindrances to losing weight can be poor past conditioning. Perhaps as a child you were not taught to feed yourself correctly. It may be that you were often given too much, or you may have been taught that food was scarce and you never had enough. Maybe you were told to always clear your plate; maybe you were given sweets as a reward or if you were upset. These examples of bad teaching and poor learning often become embedded in your unconscious thoughts and cause problems later in life.

This chapter is probably the most important in this book, so spend plenty of time working on the following techniques that will help to free you from negative associations and bad habits. The three main releasing techniques are the releasing negative conditioning technique, the parts technique, and the using positive affirmations technique. Run through each of them, and, if possible, use a combination of each to release every aspect of poor eating habits and negative associations with food. However, it is also fine to just use the technique that you prefer to achieve this aim.

No More Using Food as a Reward

It is a common occurrence nowadays for adults to "treat" themselves to something sweet and fattening—like candy or desserts—because they have done something good, have worked hard, or are upset. They "reward" themselves just as their parents rewarded them years ago. Most people are blissfully unaware they are running on programming from the past.

Make a conscious choice now to never use food or drink as a reward, as a treat, or for comfort.

They simply justify their indulgences because they are feeling pleased with themselves or feeling low.

In fact, eating for comfort and satisfaction is a common problem. It doesn't make sense to clog your system with chocolate as a reward. Overweight people will often say they "comfort eat" or see food as a reward. Make a conscious choice now to never use food or drink as a reward, as a treat, or for comfort. Make this choice resolute and clear. If you have done something you are proud of or you want to treat yourself, buy yourself some new clothes or reward yourself in an entirely positive way. You can now take comfort in the fact that you are taking control of your eating habits. This is far more rewarding and satisfying.

Releasing the Need to Comfort Eat Technique

CLOSE YOUR EYES and take a few slow deep breaths. Now affirm to yourself that you take great comfort and satisfaction that you are in control of your eating habits. State the following affirmations over and over in a slow, rhythmical chant, believing they are a reality as you say them:

- ➤ I release the need for sweet and fattening food.
- ➤ I love being in control of my eating habits.
- ➤ I deserve to be fit and healthy.

It is funny how food and drink habits can become so ingrained, or even customary. I grew up in England, and we Brits have brainwashed ourselves into believing a cup of tea solves most of life's problems. This has been passed down from previous generations. I can still hear my grandmother saying, "Have a cup of tea, love, and then you'll feel better." Bless her!

Most other nations think it is bizarre that the British drink so much tea. But tea has associations of comfort anchored within our national psyche. Tea in moderation is fine, but you need to become aware of any such associations that you may have with unhealthy food or drinks. Is there any particular fattening food or drink that you were taught was a treat or a comfort? Take a moment to think about this and create an awareness of any food or drink that you view as special because of your conditioning. You must use the banishing unhealthy food technique in Chapter 7 to help you break free of any strong attachments to specific foods. This is very important. If you have an unhealthy connection to chocolate, French fries, or other fattening food, you must free yourself from this connection and aim to create an indifference to it. This can be done easily with this reprogramming technique.

> "A man too busy to take care of his health is like a mechanic too busy to take care of his tools."
> —Spanish Proverb

Emotional Causes of Poor Eating Habits

Negative emotions can sometimes trigger poor eating habits. This is why a holistic approach to weight loss is so important—you need to release all underlying problems. In some cases people push down their emotions and overeat instead of dealing with their problems. The actual act of eating can take the mind off the fact we are sad or angry in the same way that the alcoholic drowns his or her sorrows with liquor. If you have ever tried to deal with emotional worries with food, you need to become aware of why you do this and break that habit. A little self-analysis can help. Ask yourself if you ever overeat the wrong type of foods because of an emotional cause.

Eating, grazing, or even bingeing often can be the result of unconsciously pushing down emotions. Eating temporarily helps us forget our troubles. The person who eats a whole tub of ice cream in front of the TV may be blocking out the sadness of a lost relationship or a fight with a relative. The person who grabs a bag of chips might be pushing down frustration or anger rather than expressing it to the appropriate person. Then there is the person who regularly indulges in snacks and beer in front of the TV rather than facing up to a weight problem and deteriorating health. As a child maybe these people were not taught boundaries or positive ways of dealing with problems. There is a theory that those who crave a lot of sweet foods have lost the sweetness in their lives. If these examples are similar to any of your bad habits, you need to get to the bottom of each one and deal with the causes.

Poor eating helps to suppress your real feelings, but this artificial comfort eating is very damaging in the long term and will only exacerbate problems. If you numb yourself with fattening foods and do not deal with your real feelings, the negative cycle will continue. You need to break out of any such destructive patterns by dealing with the underlying causes so that you can then focus on creating a healthy mind and body. You will feel so much better when you do this. Make a point of being proactive when problems arise and avoid any poor eating or drinking habits at these times.

Freeing Yourself from Poor Conditioning

You are going to learn many techniques to help free you from poor conditioning from your past. If you learned poor eating habits, you can *unlearn* them and create positive patterns instead. In the same way that a whole nation has created a psychological belief that a cup of tea will relax them, you can start to program yourself in a positive way to create good habits.

Water is the most precious drink, and when you can get into the habit of drinking lots of it, you will notice many benefits. Water flushes away toxins, improves your complexion, helps with digestion, and can replace the need for snacking between meals. Try the loving the taste of pure fresh water technique with the goal that a healthy drink of water will now replace any snacking habits in between meals.

Now the thought of drinking water in place of eating dessert or candy may not sound very appealing, but

Loving the Taste of Pure Fresh Water Technique

CLOSE YOUR EYES and take a few slow deep breaths. Center your mind and repeat the following affirmation to yourself. State the following affirmation over and over in a slow rhythmical chant.

➤ I love the taste of pure fresh water.

As you affirm this, imagine the crystal-clear water pouring into your mouth, bringing a strong feeling of refreshment. *Taste* the water in your mouth and really enjoy the *sensation* of drinking it. Repeat this affirmation and visualization regularly.

After the first time you do this affirmation, drink a fresh glass of bottled or filtered water and notice how good it tastes. Use this visualization a few more times and you will be well on the way to creating a healthy habit that will last a lifetime.

remember you are working on a deep level to create new beliefs that you will respond to automatically. You are bypassing the ego-driven, conscious intellect and creating a new deep-rooted belief that feeds your conscious mind so that you will think that you *love* the taste of water and the thought of desserts or candy will seem unappealing. When you create a strong visualization that you love drinking water instead of snacking, your mind will soon accept this reality.

> *If you learned poor eating habits, you can unlearn them and create new positive patterns of behavior instead.*

You Are Your Own Best Therapist

At this point you need to be your own therapist. If you have poor eating habits in adulthood that you know relate to your childhood, you need to self-analyze and find the cause of the problem. It is not about blame, as parents often make these mistakes with their children inadvertently. Maybe *they* also had poor past conditioning and didn't know any better. Whatever the case, you are now going to break that cycle and take back control of your eating habits.

If you overeat, comfort eat, indulge in too much sweet food, eat too late, or snack between meals, you need to stop these negative patterns. There is always a reason why bad habits begin, so just take a moment to focus on any such eating problems now. Is there anything in your past that has caused you to have poor eating habits now? You will know best here because each person will have personal reasons for his or her eating habits.

Take time here to analyze where the cause of the poor conditioning began. You need to develop a greater understanding of where the problems lie. It is important to make sure you release anything holding you back. Once you clarify these problem areas in your conscious awareness, you can focus on them by using the writing exercises that follow.

These exercises will help you identify why you overeat and understand the root causes of the problem. If you answer yes to any of the questions, close your eyes and let your mind go back to the time when these patterns started so that you can analyze the root causes. If you are not exactly sure of the origins of the problems, close your eyes, take a few deep breaths, and ask your inner mind when the problems may have started. If still nothing comes to mind, affirm that your unconscious mind will give you the answer when the time is right. It may be that a day or two later the answer pops into your head. If this is the case, then come back to this section and write down the answer.

Do you overeat for comfort or to feel temporarily happy or content? What do you think might have first triggered this problem behavior pattern in your past?

Do you overeat when you feel stressed or emotional? What was it that first triggered this problem behavior pattern?

_____

_____

_____

_____

Do you overeat out of boredom? What was it that first triggered this problem behavior pattern?

_____

_____

_____

_____

Do you overeat because you are unhappy with other areas of your life? What was it that first triggered this problem behavior pattern?

_____

_____

_____

_____

Do you overeat because of a negative past experience? What was it that first triggered this problem behavior pattern?

_____

_____

_____

_____

Do you overeat because of other people (e.g., because friends, coworkers, or relatives) encourage you? When did this problem behavior pattern begin?

_____

_____

_____

_____

Do you overeat because you feel safe or protected by being overweight? What was it that first triggered this problem behavior pattern?

_____

_____

_____

Do you overeat out of a lack of discipline or greed? What was it that first triggered this problem behavior pattern?

_____

_____

_____

_____

List any other reasons you might have for overeating along with the root causes.

_____

_____

_____

_____

Now that you are aware of the origins of the problems holding you back, you can work on the causes by using the releasing negative conditioning and the parts techniques to free yourself from the causes forever.

The releasing negative conditioning technique will help you release destructive eating patterns. This technique can be very effective for breaking lifelong negative habits. Learn the technique well before you begin and use all of your senses—visual, auditory, feeling, taste, and smell—when following the steps.

Releasing Negative Conditioning Technique

TAKE A MOMENT to get comfortable, close your eyes, and focus on breathing. Take a few slow deep breaths, and allow your mind to become still and quiet and your body to relax.

When you feel pleasantly relaxed, focus on an eating issue that is a problem and think of the root cause of that problem. Go back in time to when the problem began, and imagine you are viewing it from a distance as though you are watching a video.

Now you are watching yourself at the time of the start of this problem. You can see clearly why the problem started. You understand the reason this pattern started, but you are going to let it go now because it is no longer helping you. Feel as though you are letting go of the cause of the problem. Imagine yourself releasing the cause. Put your feelings into letting it go forever.

As you let go, imagine the picture turns to black and white. Soon the whole picture fades until the screen becomes blank. You now feel very detached from the cause of the problem, as though it is no longer a part of you, just a fading memory. Imagine the old negative patterns have completely disappeared.

Feel a strong sense of well-being inside, as though you have let go of a burden, something you no longer need or want. You feel very secure in yourself now and you affirm to yourself:

- I am free of the old negative pattern of behavior.
- I love being fit and healthy.

Take a moment to absorb these affirmations into your mind. Repeat them slowly a dozen or so times. As the affirmations resonate inside you, imagine the video screen flashing to life once again. This time you see a bright clear picture of yourself in the present. The picture now shows that you are completely free of the old problem. The old poor eating pattern has gone, and you have a positive new pattern in its place.

You are back in control and you notice how good you feel. The picture is clear and colorful, and you realize it is up-to-date and the new healthy way you will now cope in this situation.

Take a moment to absorb the positive new images and feelings. Then, when you are ready, slowly count to five and open your eyes. When you do this, it is important to affirm that every part of you is back in the present, while the underlying problem that was causing your unhealthy eating habits is no longer a part of you—gone forever.

Be clear about your aim and practice the technique many times. If after the first time you use the technique you still have the problem, then repeat it again and again until the problem disappears. You are in effect learning how to rewire your brain and erase destructive conditioning. Some old programs can be harder to shift than others and may need more attention.

Freeing Yourself from Comfort or Stress Eating

Why when you are under pressure or feel stressed would you want to do something that will make you feel even worse? Why do people compound their anxiety by eating fattening food that will make them feel worse about themselves? Odd, isn't it? If as a child you were taught that a brownie is a little treat or were given sweets after a trauma of some kind, the belief that certain food is comforting can become lodged in your psyche. However, these patterns can easily be changed by using the following technique.

Parts Technique

CLOSE YOUR EYES and begin to breathe slowly and deeply in through your nose and out through your mouth in a steady circular rhythm. Think of nothing but your breathing. Aim to create a feeling of complete relaxation through your breathing and mental focus.

When you feel centered and relaxed, imagine the child part of you who was given sweets or some other food as a treat. Maybe you were given cookies after you did something worthy or were comforted with sweets after you suffered an accident or trauma. Maybe the food was a comfort at the time and seemed nice. Imagine the child part of you who was treated or comforted in this way. Take time to do this.

Now, clear your mind for a few seconds and then imagine another part of you—the informed adult part of you who wants to break free from comfort or stress eating. Take a second to connect with this part of you.

Bring both parts of you together and begin a dialogue. Imagine the adult part of you explaining to your child part that it isn't necessary to eat fattening food when feeling stressed or anxious. Explain that it is possible to break free of this old habit forever. Take time to go into detail and make the dialogue specific to your problem, covering all the reasons why you comfort or stress eat.

Once both parts of you are in agreement that they will not eat when they feel stressed or anxious, you can move on. When both parts are resolute in their united aim to maintain a healthy eating lifestyle, then imagine in your mind's eye the two parts merging together to become one whole.

Imagine this whole part becoming absorbed back into your body. Draw it back into your consciousness, and accept on every level you are free of any need to comfort or stress eat.

Once you are familiar with this technique you can compound it by repeating these affirmations:

- ⌐ I am free of comfort eating.
- ⌐ I now cope with anxiety and stress in positive new ways.
- ⌐ I am in control of my eating habits.
- ⌐ My healthy lifestyle brings me great comfort.

Take a moment to really absorb these positive new beliefs and feelings, and then when you are ready, slowly count to three and open your eyes. When you do this, it is important to affirm that every part of you is back in the present.

Letting go of negative beliefs under self-hypnosis can work wonders. The parts technique will help you release any destructive programming that may be causing you to comfort or stress eat. It is slightly different than the releasing negative conditioning technique. Look at which of the two scripts most addresses your specific needs. You can use both scripts or just one.

Affirmations to Overcome Negative Conditioning

The use of affirmations alone can release negative conditioning. Clearing out negative conditioning and then installing new positive beliefs with affirmations that apply specifically to you will help you achieve long-term success. You are working from the inside out, and when the "inner you" is programmed correctly, your new healthy lifestyle will become second nature and never again will you battle with your weight.

Reprogramming your thoughts is the best way to take control of your weight because you are not asked to think about food. Instead, you are focusing your mind on specific aims and allowing your inner self to assimilate a new way of thinking from which you will respond automatically.

On the CD are some affirmations to help you release negative conditioning. However, those affirmations are generalized, and this is why you need to focus on the areas that may have specifically held *you* back. Create your own personalized affirmations and use the self-hypnosis techniques to release this negative conditioning forever. As you work through whatever negative conditioning may have previously held you back, evaluate how you feel about it afterward. When you no longer need to reward yourself with food or sweets or to clear your plate at every meal—or whatever your particular problem is—then you are ready to move on.

When you reprogram yourself using your affirmations, you will be amazed at how your circumstances improve. The discipline here is working on yourself and being creative with this inner work.

The following are examples of affirmations to help release poor conditioning. You will need to create your own affirmations that best suit your aims. Get yourself into a relaxed and centered state and then repeat your affirmations slowly and steadily with total belief as you say them. Affirm your releasing affirmations regularly until you feel you have let go of any negative conditioning.

- I release my old negative conditioning about food.
- I release any need to comfort eat.
- I release any desire to overindulge with sickly sweet, fattening food.
- I release any need to overeat.

Add a few of your own affirmations, but at this stage they must only be releasing affirmations similar to the examples above. It is important you take one step at a time and only move on when you have completed each process.

Remember to make your affirmations completely unambiguous and entirely positive.

Creating Positive Affirmations

Once you feel that you have overcome poor conditioning, you are ready to develop your new positive affirmation program. The releasing affirmations help you let go of poor conditioning and release negative behavior patterns, whereas the positive affirmations help create new patterns of behavior. It is important to finish your releasing affirmation sessions *before* beginning the following positive affirmation sessions because you must focus on one exclusive goal at a time when you are working on yourself. For example, plan to spend a week working on releasing negative conditioning with affirmations and the other releasing techniques; then spend the following week working on installing positive new affirmations. Set a clear schedule for yourself that suits your needs.

Positive affirmations will help you overwrite old data that are no longer serving you. Your unconscious mind believes exactly what you tell it. It won't get emotional about your affirmations or criticize them (criticism takes place in the conscious mind). When you repeat your affirmations in a deeply relaxed state, your unconscious mind will accept the suggestions as a reality. You will then begin to respond to the new programming in your daily life without thinking about it. Keep blasting your positive affirmations deeply into your unconscious mind and you will be amazed at the progress you make.

Again you will need to create your own affirmations, but feel free to add any of the example affirmations included here to your own list. Acknowledge that you will get into the habit of affirming your phrases many times a day.

Add your own positive affirmations below, making sure they are in the present tense and in the first person. They must also be unambiguous and entirely positive.

It is easy to acquire the affirmation habit, and it is something you can do at any time. For example, in the shower or on car journeys, get into the habit of turning off the radio and repeating your affirmations instead. Make the whole positive programming thing a part of your everyday life. Most people fail to succeed because

Using Positive Affirmations Technique

GET INTO A relaxed and centered state to begin. When you state your affirmations, say them as though they are a reality now and use imagery and your feelings to turbo-charge the affirmations and make them real. Say each one ten or more times slow and steady, similar to a mantra.

- I love being in control of my eating habits.
- I eat smaller amounts of healthy food.
- I love the taste of pure fresh water.
- I love to exercise and keep fit.
- My self-esteem grows stronger and stronger.
- I remain a healthy eater forever.

they are half-hearted; but if you state your intent clearly and work diligently toward it, you will reach your goal. Cultivate these good habits and build them into your daily routines. *You will be amazed at how quickly things can change when you are resonating with these new beliefs.*

The more you work at your reprogramming, the quicker you will achieve your target weight. Remember to enjoy the journey—creating positive mental states on a regular basis can be fun and empowering in many ways.

Other Possible Solutions

Once the negative associations have gone, you can be free of the destructive conditioning that held you back in the past. It then becomes so much easier to embrace the healthy lifestyle. You will feel liberated and free of the unconscious urge to self-destruct.

If you have a number of problems that relate to poor past conditioning, I suggest you continue working with these techniques for each problem because you need to be completely free of any destructive past eating issues. Work through the releasing techniques as many times as you need to, until there is nothing else holding you back.

There is a wide range of alternative therapies and treatments available today that are good at healing the root causes of problems. I am a big fan of treatments such as homeopathy and kinesiology, which often work well in conjunction with hypnotherapy. Without having used many of these types of treatments in the past, I believe I would still be stuck in patterns of behavior that were preventing me from progressing in life. Some people will respond better to certain therapies than to others, so try a few and see which ones work best for you. There is always a solution out there; all you need is the desire to overcome your problems.

Life can be like a horse race where each horse carries a different weight on his back. Some people's start in life is fraught with difficulties, and they carry more weight than those who have had a loving, nurturing, stable upbringing. But even though some of us carry extra baggage, with a little knowledge and determination we can overcome that handicap and succeed in our aims. It comes down to how much we want it and how much energy we put into achieving it.

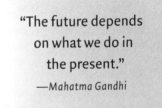

"The future depends on what we do in the present."
—Mahatma Gandhi

You may want to include your own affirmations with your preferred releasing technique to free yourself from your own specific constraints from the past. Do not underestimate this work because it underpins everything you are going to achieve. Clearing out old negative conditioning is crucial in order to develop new healthy eating patterns.

Every good therapist will adapt techniques to suit their clients. If a certain technique doesn't work well for you, use another suitable technique in this book to get rid the problem. You may even adapt the techniques for your specific aim. In effect you are learning to become your own therapist. There is also much on the CD to help you in these areas, but it is good to do your own work and become self-sufficient.

For the majority, the self-hypnosis and releasing techniques in this chapter will be sufficient to help you move forward. However, if destructive past programming has been a major problem, you may want to consider a series of one-to-one sessions with a good therapist. I have included some information on what to look for in a therapist in Chapter 6.

6

Building
Powerful Self-Esteem

Be honest with yourself and put your

energy into making positive personal

changes that improve the quality of your

life. Being overweight is not an illness; it is

merely an accumulation of bad habits.

THERE IS often a link between weight problems and low self-esteem. The reasons may be complex, but people with low self-esteem often seek comfort or solace in food. Or, they may lack the discipline needed to look after themselves and have low self-esteem as a result. However, with a little effort your self-esteem can be improved.

Building Self-Esteem

In most cases our feelings of self-worth are formed through our learned experiences in childhood. If you weren't encouraged to love and respect yourself, then you probably suffer low self-esteem. The first rule of learning to love and respect yourself is to banish negative self-talk from your vocabulary.

Whatever you repeatedly affirm will become self-fulfilling.

Self-criticism is extremely destructive. Your unconscious mind accepts the things you say unconditionally. If you are forever berating yourself for being stupid or foolish, all you are doing is programming yourself to feel that way. Remember, whatever you repeatedly affirm will become self-fulfilling.

After eliminating self-criticism from your inner dialogue, you can learn to love and respect yourself more by focusing on your successes. Being a good parent to your children is a major success in life and all too often very overlooked. Being kind, loving, compassionate, and generous are also wonderful traits that most people possess. If you have ever won or achieved anything, however small, don't be afraid to praise yourself. Maybe you are doing well at work, or you have achieved a personal goal. Always look at what you have achieved, acknowledge it, and be proud of yourself. There is nothing wrong with praising and being proud of yourself—it is something you should embrace. Use the learning to love and

SELF-ESTEEM TIP: ELIMINATE NEGATIVE SELF-TALK

Never ever speak negatively to yourself. This can be so destructive. If you repeat something often enough, your unconscious mind will soon accept it as a reality. So, if you often berate yourself by calling yourself stupid or useless, you are actually programming yourself in a very negative way. You will then unconsciously respond to that negative programming and actually create situations for yourself that make you feel stupid or useless.

Remember the computer analogy—what you program in is what will come back out. The human mind is exactly like that, so from now on you must never vocally or internally say (or even think) negative things about yourself. I know this is not always easy if you have had a lifetime of negative conditioning and your self-esteem is low, but you need to start fresh from this moment on. By reprogramming your "computer" with positive beliefs about yourself, over time you will build more confidence and self-esteem. It is a case of "fake it until you make it."

From now on view your mistakes and errors as things that will teach you something. Look for the lesson in the error, but do not punish or berate yourself. Sometimes we learn the biggest lessons through our mistakes. The key is to learn the lesson so you don't make the same mistake again and retain your self-belief by maintaining a positive internal dialogue.

respect yourself technique regularly to help you build your self-esteem.

Learning to Love and Respect Yourself Technique

LEARN TO LOVE yourself completely, faults and all. When you truly love and respect yourself, you open yourself up to being loved and respected by others. Cultivate the habit of loving yourself by acknowledging your achievements and focusing on your good points.

Close your eyes, take a few deep breaths, and relax. Take a few moments to clear away any unwanted thoughts and let your mind become still. Then focus on all the little things that you have achieved in your life—any good work you have done, any good friendships you have cultivated, anything you have won or been praised for. Keep your focus on all the positives in your life and feel really good about yourself as you do so.

Enhance and even exaggerate all the feelings and images by making them big, bright, and very clear. Be proud of yourself as you do this and repeat the following affirmations:

- I love and respect myself.
- I am proud of myself.
- My self-esteem is strong.

Repeat the affirmations over and over like a slow mantra, saying the words with total belief and real conviction. This is a good exercise to put very strong feelings into, but make sure you remain deeply relaxed at the same time. Draw these words deep inside you so they really resonate with you.

Continue this technique regularly over a number of days until you feel your self-esteem growing strong.

As your self-esteem grows, your desire to improve the quality of your life and be healthy will also grow stronger. When your self-esteem is strong, you will only want to do things that are good for your well-being. You simply won't *want* to load your body up with fattening food, vegetate in front of the TV every night, or let your body become bloated and out of shape. Instead you will have an inner desire that drives you to make positive changes and improve all aspects of your life. You will also naturally gravitate toward other people who believe in themselves and who have positive aims.

When you build strong self-esteem and a disciplined approach toward your eating and exercise habits, it is easy to connect with like-minded people. Your outer life is often a reflection of your inner thoughts and feelings. So look around you. If you don't like what you see, make the necessary changes from within and things will soon change around you. You have the free will to make changes, and with a little effort and discipline you will do just that.

If there are issues from your past connected to weight control that have held you back, make a vow to yourself to achieve your weight loss goal in spite of the past. Don't hold on to any anger against those who contributed to your low self-esteem and weight problems. This is a waste of your energy. If you believe other people have caused you to suffer and you hold on to the anger, those same people still have power over you. All this anger does is continue to hold *you* back.

> *Your outer life is often a reflection of your inner thoughts and feelings.*

Use the releasing techniques in Chapter 5 if you need to let go of any negativity or anger relating to the past. If you need further help, seek out a well-qualified hypnotherapist. When seeking out a hypnotherapist for a one-on-one session, call a few and find someone you feel comfortable with. Check that the person's qualifications are from a well-established body, and ask for references and proof of insurance if you feel the need.

> "Courage is the mastery of fear, not the absence of fear."
> —Mark Twain

Good therapy is all about dynamics between the therapist and client. So finding a therapist who inspires you and who can get to the root of any problem is the key to successful therapy.

No matter what, never give up on letting go of negativity and anger because hanging on to negative emotions will only slow *your* progress. The positive self-image technique will help your self-image. Once again, you are aiming to program your mind with a new belief, which it will automatically respond to.

Positive Self-Image Technique

CLOSE YOUR EYES. Breathe slowly and deeply until your mind is still and you feel very relaxed. Then imagine yourself as you want to be. Create a picture of the perfect you standing in front of you, full of confidence and self-belief. See the confident way this self-assured you stands and how you hold yourself. Make the picture very positive, bright, and clear.

Now, step into your perfect self and imagine you are looking out through your own eyes. Connect with the positive feelings and notice how good you feel in your perfect self. Amplify the positive feelings, and affirm they will stay with you in your everyday life.

Practice this technique regularly, especially at times when your confidence and self-esteem need a boost.

Positive Modeling

As human beings we often seek to validate our behavior weaknesses and bad habits. It is frequently the case that people choose friends who have similar unhealthy habits because it allows them to feel okay about their own behaviors. If you are twenty-five pounds overweight and you have friends who are forty pounds overweight, it can be easy to justify your excesses by saying, "I'm not as bad as so and so."

Now I'm not saying you should dump all your overweight or unhealthy friends! But don't judge yourself against others who are weak-willed and content to stay stuck. Rather you must aspire to modeling yourself after people who are fit and healthy if that is what you really want.

> "Nothing can stop a person with the right mental attitude from achieving their goal; nothing on earth can help a person with the wrong mental attitude."
>
> —Thomas Jefferson

The brief Neuro-Linguistic Programming (NLP) modeling technique will help you learn to absorb and assimilate the same qualities held by someone who inspires you. Neuro-Linguistic Programming is a therapeutic tool for effective communication, goal setting, influencing, accelerated learning, and behavior modification. It can help you model your behavior on a positive example. It is as though you are absorbing the habits of the person in question and then importing these positive characteristics into your own consciousness.

Imagine a friend, relative, or acquaintance you know who eats healthily, exercises regularly, and has a body shape and size that you aspire to. If you can't think of anyone who fits the bill, imagine a famous super-fit athlete whom you admire.

When someone comes to mind, focus on this person as a model for your approach to weight loss and fitness. Imagine his or her healthy eating plans and fitness routines, and embrace this person's positive habits for your own aims. Read the NLP modeling script through a few times until you know what to do, and then practice this technique whenever you need inspiration.

Neuro-Linguistic Programming Modeling for Weight Loss Technique

CLOSE YOUR EYES and allow yourself to become comfortable. Breathe very slowly and deeply, in through your nose and out through your mouth. Make each breath long and deep, and relax more and more with every slow breath exhaled.

Now, focus on someone who is very fit and healthy and who inspires you. Preferably it should be a person you know and see fairly often, but if no one comes to mind focus on a famous athlete. It must be a person you admire for being *very* fit and healthy, not someone who is *reasonably* fit and healthy. Set a high goal for this technique.

Take a moment to see this person in your mind's eye, and focus on his or her level of health and fitness. Just focus on the qualities and everything that you like about this person. Take a moment to feel very inspired.

Now imagine that all of these qualities are becoming part of you. Feel as though you are drawing this person's determination and discipline deep inside yourself. Imagine you are absorbing and assimilating the same very positive, single-minded attitude toward your health and well-being. Make these traits a part of you now.

Next, visualize yourself achieving your fitness goal with the same self-belief and determination as the person you admire. You are in control of your weight now and determined to become and remain fit, toned, and healthy in the same way this person has. Take a moment to focus on this. Be creative and use all of your senses when you visualize yourself expressing the new characteristics that will help you to achieve and maintain a high level of fitness.

Take all the time you need to do this. When you are ready to finish, allow your mind to clear and slowly count from one to three. Open your eyes and come back to full waking consciousness.

Be creative when you use this technique and practice it regularly!

One thing to note is that if the person you are modeling ever goes off the rails and gains weight, this will not happen to you because you are modeling only his or her positive traits.

Banishing Negativity

Don't ever let self-doubt or negativity get in your way. Negative thoughts are a part of what makes us human—the secret is not to dwell on them. Whenever you get a negative thought, just let it drift away and refocus on the positive.

Be aware of how the media can be a negative influence. Television and radio advertisers know how to manipulate you and sometimes walk a fine line with the use of mood music and persuasive language, especially in food advertising. It seems every other TV ad is either a junk food ad or an ad featuring a warm compassionate-looking actor selling drugs for illnesses that more often than not have been caused by poor eating and lack of exercise.

In magazines we see slim celebrities of all ages looking amazing. The reality is that these pictures have often been doctored or airbrushed to make the celebrities look slimmer, younger, and generally more attractive. Don't buy into this. You must never allow yourself to feel inadequate by measuring yourself against fake media images. They are an illusion. When you look after yourself through healthy eating and exercise, you will avoid much of this hype and manipulation.

When your self-esteem grows strong, it will shine through and make you more attractive. People are drawn to others who have a strong self-belief. So it is important to use the techniques in this chapter to really build up the love and respect that you feel for yourself. As your self-respect grows stronger, you will find you attract more positive people into your life and you will naturally move away from negative people who are a drain.

Clearing Negative Thoughts Technique

CLOSE YOUR EYES and practice your preferred slow deep breathing and relaxation technique, which you should be very familiar with by now. Allow your mind to go completely blank.

Every time you get an unwanted thought, imagine a large red stop sign. As soon as you see the red stop sign, imagine the thought disappearing and your mind becoming clear.

Another thought-clearing technique is to imagine a large computer screen full of data that becomes blank by hitting the delete key. Imagine that by pressing one key you can clear your mind.

You will also find it easier to let go of negative habits because you will only do things that are congruent with the way that you feel about yourself. When you feel good about yourself, you will naturally want to cultivate a more positive mind-set and have a body that is fit and healthy.

7

Healthy Eating:
Knowledge Is Power

_____

The main thing I have learned from ten
years of being a hypnotherapist is that
the mind has unlimited potential.

THIS CHAPTER is a little different from the rest of the chapters in this book, which primarily focus on using hypnotherapy and other therapeutic techniques to help you break free of poor conditioning, lose weight, and become fit and healthy. The food and drug industries are closely tied to our weight problems, and I felt it important to include this chapter to give you a greater awareness of the effect these industries have on us. With a little knowledge about how these industries operate in this modern age, you will be able to make more informed decisions when you shop. Knowledge is power, and the more you know and understand, the more control you will have over your health and well-being.

The Food and Drug Industries

The largest food and drug companies are very powerful, and in today's global economy they are driven by making profits. These food companies do not want you to become slim and healthy, even if their advertising says they do. They aim to produce and package their food products as cheaply as possible and market them as effectively as possible with the goal of maximizing their profit margins. These companies have a vested interest in people overeating cheap, low-quality food. Obviously, this doesn't apply to all food companies, but it is the case with many. Certainly the fast-food industry and food companies producing cheap processed food are guilty of this.

Most supermarket food has been flown in from all corners of the world. If buyers can purchase foods from other parts of the world more cheaply than they can locally, that is what they do. Not a lot wrong with that you might say. But to make the longer journey to the supermarket shelves means prolonging the life of the food with added sugar, salt, chemicals, and preservatives. Increasing the shelf life of food with these methods is the key to greater profits.

Because supermarkets have such buying power, they will often turn the screws on their suppliers, which has the effect of making food producers and farmers grow or raise their produce in the shortest possible time. This, in turn, involves the use of a multitude of chemicals, pesticides, herbicides, growth hormones, and so on.

People think organic food is new and are happy to pay more for it. But up until about fifty years ago, all food was organic. Why can't all food companies produce natural, untainted, chemical-free food as they once did? The answer is: they make more money from chemically altered food that has a longer shelf life. If the demand is there, food companies will continue to produce food in this way.

When you eat food that has been processed or preserved for longevity, the nutritional content of the food will be minimal and your body will not recognize the chemically enhanced food. This type of diet can create false hunger and imbalances in the body. Conversely, when you eat highly nutritional, quality food, you feed your body with the right vitamins, nutrients, and minerals. You will also eat less because you are giving your body what it needs and properly satisfying your natural hunger.

Imagine if every man, woman, and child had a very lean, sugar-free, chemical-free, healthy diet and combined it with daily exercise. The big drug companies would soon be out of business. Their market would disappear because people would no longer be falling sick in such large numbers. They would have no one to sell their drugs to. A fit and healthy population is their worse-case scenario. It is easy to see why these powerful, influential companies so desperately want people to stay fat and unhealthy. The scary fact is that they need people to remain sick, overweight, and unhealthy, and for far too long they have succeeded.

To avoid becoming another sick statistic who then gets caught in the drug peddlers' web, all you have to

> "Let food be thy medicine and medicine be thy food."
> —Hippocrates

do is eat healthily and exercise regularly. If you ask me, it is not really a difficult choice to make. Do it now. For the sake of your family and yourself, make a vow to take that healthy option every time. How great to think that you are creating a lifestyle in which producers of low-quality food and drug companies with vested interests can't mess with your health.

Don't Believe the Hype

A crucial step on your weight loss journey is knowing which foods are genuinely good for you and which are not. That means seeing beyond food marketing and public relations campaigns. Supermarkets and food companies play a big part in telling you what to eat. Often they do not have your best interests at heart, so finding the truth about healthy food is crucial. When I discovered the way in which most food is produced, packaged, and marketed, I quickly changed the way I shopped. I recommend some great books on this subject in the Resources.

Through the years there have been countless TV ads that have created the false illusion that a certain food or drink is good for you when, in fact, it is not. The government is slowly recognizing this and proposing the banning of some of the more sinister unhealthy food and drink ads, especially those aimed at children. High-sugar foods are often perceived as being a little treat. In reality they are unhealthy, fattening, and no good for you at all. So why do people see sweets or chocolate as a harmless treat or something special? Because they have been repeatedly sold that image and manipulated into believing it.

> *Nowadays, we take in monumental amounts of sugar without even realizing it.*

Nowadays we take in monumental amounts of sugar without even realizing it because virtually everything has added sugar, often in the guise of corn syrup or glucose syrup. Processed sugar is hidden in so many different foods on our supermarket shelves. Consumers just don't realize this, nor do they understand how bad it is for them.

The only sugar we need is the natural sugar found in fruits—not the processed stuff that can lead to health problems. Get into the habit of reading the ingredients on food labels. Check carefully what the "healthy food" item you have been drawn to actually contains. It is not easy to buy foods that are *genuinely* free of chemicals, preservatives, additives, and processed sugars. With many foods being sold as healthy when this is not the case, you need to be more vigilant when you shop.

> "In the struggle for survival, the fittest win out at the expense of their rivals because they succeed in adapting themselves best to their environment."
>
> —Charles Darwin

The manipulation that goes on today is scary, but as I have said, knowledge is power. Armed with knowledge you can make informed decisions. You are not going to buy the "healthy slimming" product full of additives and chemicals, which is actually designed to make you eat *more*. You are not going to take the drugs that supposedly help you with an illness that has been caused by poor diet and foods loaded with sugar and preservatives.

You can avoid these scams and reclaim your power by eating healthily and exercising regularly. Be smarter than the marketers, and take personal responsibility for your health and well-being. If you cut out sugar and foods loaded with chemicals, additives, and preservatives, you will be giving your health the best tonic possible. You won't need to rely on doctors and drugs to deal with ill-

FOOD BUYING TIP

When you shop, make sure that you only buy foods that support your goal. Banish any unhealthy food or drink from your shopping cart. If you are a mother and buying food for your family, then make these changes for them as well. If that seems difficult, use your newly learned persuasion skills to help your family make healthy lifestyle changes. If you pitch it right, your children will go along with you. They love positive changes and will respond if you frame it well.

nesses caused by low-nutritional food. By eating healthy nutritious food, you will be taking back control of your eating and your health. It is as simple as that.

Creating Positive Eating Habits

In August 2006 the International Association of Agricultural Economists announced, "The world now has more overweight people than hungry ones. There are more than a billion overweight people in the world and 800 million who are undernourished." The association added that worldwide hunger is slowly declining while obesity is rapidly spreading.

We live in an age where for the vast majority of people in the Western world, food is in abundant supply. We have access to many varieties of food from around the world. People now enjoy eating more than ever—and spend more time thinking about it. When we go out for meals, the choices of restaurants and food types are numerous, and so our palatable needs and wants are often given a lot of attention. For the first time in history, we don't just eat to live, we also eat for pleasure.

A common problem is that when we eat and enjoy a meal we sometimes don't want it to end. Restaurants will frequently offer three large servings or more and round it off with dessert and coffee. Whenever you dine out, try avoiding these pitfalls by having just one main course and eating slowly. If you have an appetizer, choose something very light such as a salad with a naturally low-fat organic dressing or soup without bread. After your main meal and before you even consider eating more, allow your food to digest for at least fifteen minutes. When you use these strategies, your initial hunger will have been satisfied and you won't want to eat anything more. You will have given your body what it needs—no more, no less.

In this day when food is available in abundance, another good habit to get into is to be thankful for your food. Older generations often said prayers at family meal-times. This was because in times gone by, when food was scarce, having a wholesome meal was considered a blessing. We should all be grateful for the fact that we can eat three healthy meals a day. Never take that for granted; be thankful for each meal and enjoy it.

When you eat, be aware of the taste and texture of your food. Familiarizing your sense of smell with the

HEALTHY EATING TIP

Get into the habit of eating slowly and chewing your food well. This should be your golden rule from now on, one you cultivate consciously. Eating slowly and chewing your food longer serves to satisfy your taste buds more completely, enabling you to feel satiated quickly. It also helps your body digest the food more easily.

Adopt this habit whenever you eat. And remember, as soon as you feel full, stop eating even if there is food left on your plate. If you were taught "you must clear your plate," forget it. That old conditioning no longer applies to you now.

food before you eat can also help with digestion. When you eat three meals a day and eat slowly and consciously, you will enjoy your meals and feel more satisfied after each one.

Avoid eating too late because you are less likely to be active after your evening meal. There is an old saying that to get the maximum from our food we should eat like a king for breakfast, a prince at lunchtime, and a pauper for dinner. There is good logic behind that saying.

TIPS FOR DEVELOPING NEW EATING HABITS

Follow these guidelines for the next twenty-one days, and they will become new eating habits that will stay with you forever.

- Stick to three main meals a day and drink plenty of water throughout the day.
- Avoid eating heavy meals late in the evening.
- Eat slowly and chew your food well.
- Give your full attention to your food by eating consciously.
- Stop eating as soon as you feel full.

When you eat, give your full attention to your food and avoid doing anything else like reading or watching TV. All functions of the human body trigger chemical reactions in your brain, and when you eat your brain produces a signal to indicate when you are full. By eating slowly, chewing your food well, and eating consciously, the signal from your body to your brain that you are full is much clearer.

As I discussed earlier, people often overeat because of poor conditioning or bad habits. One of the oldest—and worst—eating habits is the need for dessert after a full meal. Nutritionally, your body has had what it needs, so why then add a cake or a brownie? This habit goes back

> **"Gluttony kills more than the sword."**
> —Old Proverb

to "treating ourselves." Having a little treat after dinner, like many families do, is an old habit. In truth, you are harming your health when you indulge too often in this way. The "treating" comes from a time when food was scarce and people would have a sweet as a treat after dinner. You don't need to do this anymore, even if it's been a family tradition. You must avoid any such habits and learn to "treat" yourself in new positive ways. *You are not "treating" yourself if you are creating an overweight and sluggish body.*

Even if you are out to dinner with others and everyone else orders a dessert, you don't have to. Dare to be different! Say, "No, thanks" to dessert. Not because your ego is driving you or because you want to make a grand statement for others to witness. You are simply choosing not to overindulge. Even if your arm is twisted, enjoy saying, "No, thanks, not for me." And smile as you say it, enjoying the feeling of being in control.

Avoiding Addictive Food

Did you know that junk food, sweets, and chocolate frequently have additives in them to make you crave them? You are not actually craving the food itself but the addictive additive content. Have you ever avoided chocolate for a long period and never even thought about it, but then eaten some and started craving it the next day?

In February 2003, the highly respected *New Scientist* printed the article "Burgers on the Brain: Can You Really Get Addicted to Fast Food?" It states how research strongly suggests that some fast foods "can act on the brain the same way as nicotine and heroin." The article went on to suggest "the need for a health warning or other appropriate informational notice to customers who might not otherwise be aware of this important new information."

This problem was the focus of the film *Supersize Me*, in which the protagonist ate only McDonald's food three times a day for thirty days. A few days into this regime he had feelings of depression, lethargy, and headaches, which were relieved only by his next McDonald's meal. He also experienced mood swings, sexual dysfunction, and liver damage. After twenty days his doctor told him to quit because his liver was becoming more pickled by the day and he was putting himself at serious risk of heart disease. Despite the warnings he continued, and when he did stop eating junk food after thirty days, he went into depressive states and suffered withdrawal symptoms similar to alcoholics or drug addicts when they go cold turkey. Scary!

Some people who run fast-food chains don't care about the quality of their food. Their sole aim is to make junk food as cheaply as possible and to sell it to as many people as possible. The shareholders are the ones who count. Regularly taking your children to these places is one of the worst things you possibly can do for them. I was once guilty of this. When my son was young I took him to birthday parties at fast-food chains—then I wised up.

The 80/20 Rule

Stick to three small healthy meals a day and avoid snacking between meals. It is okay on the odd occasion if you have a blowout, but do try to stick to the 80/20 rule: if 80 percent of the time you are doing the good stuff—eating well and exercising—then you can allot 20 percent of the time for guilt-free overindulgence.

You may go to a party or to dinner and drink too much or eat too much rich food. This is okay *now and again*, but don't let it disrupt your overall healthy lifestyle plan. If you ever overdo it, don't beat yourself up, just vow to get back on track the following day. Accept that you may experience the odd lapse from time to time, but affirm that it won't affect your long-term aims. Nothing runs smoothly 100 percent of the time; there will be a few ups and downs. This should not be a problem if you are focused on a long-term holistic goal.

No More Dieting or Scales

Do not use the words *diet, dieting,* or *slimming* because you probably have many negative associations with these words from past diets that failed. Banish these words from your vocabulary, replacing them with phrases like "healthy eating" and "my new healthy lifestyle."

You must also avoid weighing yourself. Everyone is different, and some people can eat healthily and exercise regularly for a couple of weeks and not see any discernible weight loss. That will not matter in the long term, and you should not get disheartened if this happens. If you don't have a scale, you can't weigh yourself.

When you let these unhealthy habits go, don't see it as if you are denying yourself. Simply think of it as looking after yourself. You are nurturing yourself by feeding your body correctly. You are getting into the habit of training yourself to take care of your health. You have probably already taught yourself to enjoy certain foods and drinks in the past—but not always for the good of your health.

Losing weight in the short term is not what this journey is about. It is irrelevant whether you lose a few pounds here and there. This is about you creating a new balanced and healthy lifestyle that you can maintain forever. When you banish unhealthy food, eat healthily instead, and exercise regularly, you will lose weight. If it doesn't happen immediately, don't let it be an issue. In the long term, you will lose weight the best possible way—slowly and steadily. Then once you reach your target weight, it will be easy to maintain because you have created a healthy new lifestyle.

Think of your weight management like a bank account. If at least 80 percent of the time you are eating healthily and exercising regularly, then in a year's time your bank account is going to be in healthy shape. I find now that whenever I have a little blip and overindulge, I am eager to work it off with a quick workout. This is because I am in control of my weight. It is a natural way of thinking now and not something I have to work at.

Training Your Mind to Dislike Fattening Foods

You can train your mind to dislike fattening foods, sweets, and unhealthy drinks and to genuinely love vegetables, fruit, and water. If you create a habit of consciously doing this, your mind will absorb and assimilate these affirmations and in time you will create a new healthy reality. You will soon find yourself reaching for mineral water instead of coffee or a soft drink *and* enjoying it!

Most people's first experience with alcohol is really a trial. Remember that taste of beer or wine when you were young? Most of us thought, *That tastes horrible, what's all the fuss about?* But because you wanted to be grown up and drink like an adult, you trained yourself to like it. It is the same with smoking. Many smokers hate their first cigarette but with perseverance and through gritted teeth grow to like it. The habit sticks, and they find they can't do without cigarettes. Bizarre, isn't it? I know because I was a smoker until I quit for good seventeen years ago.

Many smokers even brainwash themselves into believing that cigarettes make them feel better and help them relax. In truth, nicotine constricts arteries and increases adrenaline. Smoking is a stimulant. But people do relax with a cigarette because they have conditioned themselves to *believe* they will. If I told you every time you gave a gentle tug to your right earlobe you would feel very relaxed, after a while this would become a reality. You would relax every time you tugged on your ear. Your unconscious mind unquestioningly believes what you tell it—especially when you compound a belief through repetition.

When you are on a healthy eating plan, never think of it as a hardship or that you're losing something. Always focus on what it is giving you—your health and a fit body. You can learn to love healthy food and dislike junk food. It is simply a choice you can easily make. By making a conscious habit of saying to yourself that you hate junk food, your mind will eventually get the message and you will indeed end up hating junk food. So why not program your mind to dislike sugar and fattening processed food? Instead, teach yourself to love pure mineral water and nutritional, healthy food. Make that choice right now. *Think of it as a huge gift that you have this wonderful mind that you can program for your own good.*

Bad Food Reprogramming

The main thing I have learned from ten years of being a hypnotherapist is that the mind has unlimited potential. It knows no limitation. Often it is fear that stops us from living life to the fullest and fear of change that prevents us moving forward. Use the unlimited power of your mind to live the way you know is best for you—free of junk food and drink.

Nutritional Guidance and the Need to Wise Up!

One important step to take on the road to health and fitness is to wise up about the foods you eat. You need

Banishing Unhealthy Food Technique

THE FOLLOWING SCRIPT will help you train yourself to banish unhealthy foods from your diet. It is an excellent reprogramming technique for removing the desire for specific junk food and sweets from your life. Think of a single unhealthy or fattening food or drink that you would like to eradicate from your diet. This could be burgers, fries, chocolate, cookies, or any food or drink that is keeping you stuck at an unhealthy weight.

Close your eyes; take a few slow, deep breaths; and allow your mind to clear. Take a moment to go inside yourself and totally relax. When you are ready, imagine a plate full of the most putrid rotting fish (or maggots or something similar that is repulsive to you). Connect this picture in your mind's eye with the revolting smell of the fish. Hold back from gagging, but make this image and smell very real. Take a moment to do this.

When you have a clear picture and have imagined the foul smell, bring in the fattening food you want to erase from your diet and mix it up with the rotting fish. If it is chocolate, imagine the chocolate all over the fish making an even more disgusting smell. If it is a soft drink, imagine one of the fish inside a glass of that fizzy drink.

Be creative with this part of the technique; the more vivid you can make this image, the more powerful it will be. Allow a few minutes to digest this disgusting image and odor, and then allow your mind to become blank. Take a few slow breaths, slowly count to three, and open your eyes.

The next time you think about the food or drink that you mixed up with the rotting fish you will feel completely different. You will have lost any desire for that food or drink, or you may even find it quite repulsive now.

You can use this technique to systematically eradicate all bad foods and drinks from your diet. Focus on eliminating one thing at a time, and make sure you have lost all desire for it before moving on to the next food or drink you want to eradicate.

---

to know conclusively which foods are good for you and which are not. You have been bombarded by food company advertising, and you probably have many misconceptions about healthy food. For example, most people presume pasta is healthy. If it is unrefined brown pasta, then it is indeed healthy. However, if we are talking about white or even brown pasta that has been processed, then the nutritional content is just about zero. Some brands also have added sugar and can be very fattening. Bread and other carbohydrates are exactly the same; even some brown breads have been dyed and are loaded with sugar. When buying bread, rice, or pasta, always get the unrefined brown variety.

Highly refined sugars are processed into many foods, including bread, breakfast cereal, pasta, mayonnaise, peanut butter, ketchup, spaghetti sauce, and many microwave-ready meals. All of these foods should be avoided, along with most packaged and processed foods because the refining process kills the nutrients in the food. This is also the case when you microwave food. If you have a microwave, get rid of it! When you eat refined food with no nutritional content, you will be hungry more often because your body is craving nutrition. Conversely, when you eat healthy, nutritious food, you will not feel hungry between meals because your body is getting the nutrients it needs.

I also recommend buying organic food whenever possible. Organic food is chemical- and additive-free and is becoming less expensive as the demand for it increases. Budgeting a little more money to spend on good-quality food should be your number one priority when you shop. For convenience, there are more and more online organic food shops that offer home delivery services. I have an organic food delivery every week, which I find so much easier than traipsing round supermarkets looking at minute food ingredient labels. Incidentally, the reason these ingredient labels are so small is because often the food manufacturers don't want you to know what is in the food. If you knew, you probably wouldn't buy it.

> "Nothing will benefit human health and increase the chances for survival of life on Earth as much as the evolution to a vegetarian diet."
> —Albert Einstein

I am not going into much detail here about which foods are healthful and which should be avoided, because this is not what this book is about. However, if anything in these few paragraphs has been a bit of an eye-opener to you, then you need to learn more about nutrition and healthy food.

- **Choose these healthy foods:** vegetables, fruit, fish, white meat, white cheese, rye and spelt bread, unrefined brown rice, unrefined pasta, free-range eggs, butter (unsalted), natural (unsalted, unroasted) nuts, soy, live yogurt, raw unprocessed honey. Whenever possible, buy organic.

- **Avoid these foods and ingredients:** sugar, salt, white bread, white pasta, white flour, carbohydrates, brown bread and pasta that have been refined or dyed, artificial sweeteners, refined fats, fried food, yogurts loaded with sugar, cakes, cookies, potato chips, chocolate and sweets, canned food, ready meals, and so on. Also avoid anything labeled "reduced sugar" as well as most packaged food.

- **Buy healthy drinks:** Glass-bottled mineral water, 100 percent natural organic juices, organic red wine, organic herbal teas, and organic soy milk.

- **Avoid these drinks:** soft drinks, most alcohol, coffee, and processed milk.

This is by no means a definitive list, and I strongly urge you to do more research in this area. I recommend some good books on this subject in the Resources.

The bottom line is if you get the good food/bad food concept right 80 percent of the time you will be okay. If you stumble, don't allow yourself to slip back into bad habits.

8

Developing
New Habits

There is nothing as satisfying and rewarding as watching your body become toned and firm. It builds your self-respect and inspires you to live ever more healthily.

BECAUSE SO many people are overweight nowadays it can almost seem normal. It is crazy that being overweight should be regarded as the norm. In this day and age when food is in abundance, you need to make a little more effort to keep the pounds from piling on. This chapter offers a number of weight loss and exercise suggestions and ideas for implementing them. Some will be more suitable for you than others, so use the ones that work best for you.

The Detox Option

One of the best ways to lose weight is to detox—spending a week or two consuming water, fresh juices, vegetables, fruits, and nuts. There are different types of detox plans, including ones that are strict low-calorie, fluids-only, which is acceptable if you are reasonably fit and have a week or two without much to do. However, for your first time, a detox plan that includes fluids, vegetables, fruits, and nuts would be advisable. *The Juice Master: Turbo-Charge Your Life in 14 Days* offers some great juicing advice and a well-balanced introduction to detoxification.

Detoxing is a great way to help you cleanse your system and break free of destructive eating habits or any food, alcohol, or nicotine addictions. The first few days on detox may give you an occasional headache and leave you feeling rough, but this is simply because your body is letting go of toxins—not because it is bad for you. After three days you will start to feel good, and your energy levels will increase if you are exercising regularly. After one week you will feel amazing, you will be full of energy and a few pounds lighter, and your eyes will sparkle like a film star's!

> "Our health always seems much more valuable after we lose it."
> —Anonymous

Of course, you will come across studies claiming that detoxing is a waste of time because our bodies can easily eliminate alien substances—pesticides, hormones, preservatives, and herbicides—found in many foods and drinks. Other studies will confirm the opposite—that toxic chemicals and additives in food have harmful effects on our systems.

I have my doubts about studies that "prove" chemicals in food are okay and bear no relation to the increases in the rates of cancers and other diseases. I prefer to apply my own logic and common sense rather than trust studies with vested interests behind them. From personal experience I can tell you that detoxing works. I recently spent a week on a detoxification, yoga, and meditation retreat in a remote part of Turkey. For the first three days we did not eat and drank only specially prepared juices three times a day. The ingredients of the juices were carefully planned so that we took in all the vitamins and minerals the body needs. There were thirty people on this retreat from all age groups and backgrounds, but every one of them gained great benefit from it—so much so that we collectively lost the weight of one person. The total group weight loss for the week was around 150 pounds. On top of that everyone went home full of energy.

> "The health of the people is really the foundation upon which all their happiness and all their powers as a state depend."
> —Benjamin Disraeli

If you make a decision to buy a juicer and go on a two-week detox while exercising regularly, you will look and feel fantastic at the end of it. It will kick-start your new healthy holistic lifestyle in the best possible way. For a holistic approach to detoxing it is good to exercise more, and there are a number of exercise suggestions later in this chapter. It is also advisable to reduce the amount of TV you watch during detox because you are aiming to empower yourself and create healthy new routines, so you need as few distractions as possible. You can plan a detox to suit your budget, although other than the cost of buying a juicing machine, juicing vegetables and fruit is often inexpensive.

If you are eager to make a flying start to your new healthy eating plan, why not begin with a detoxification plan during which you only drink water and fresh vegetable juices and eat fruits, nuts, and vegetables for two weeks? If you have a medical condition of any kind, you must check with your physician first. But, if you are in good health and have professional guidance, detoxing is a wonderful way to begin a new healthy lifestyle.

Some of the main benefits you will feel after a combination of detox and daily exercise include improved sleep, waking up feeling much brighter in the morning, increased energy, sparkling eyes, and softer wrinkles. You may also find minor illnesses and ailments will disappear. Another significant benefit is that after eating nothing but healthy food for two weeks you will completely lose the desire for sweet, fattening foods. Try eating a chocolate brownie after detox and it will make you want to gag.

Combining detox with a simple exercise routine will change your life in a short amount of time and get you firmly on the road to achieving health and fitness. I said earlier that it is wise to avoid losing weight too quickly. However, when you lose weight in a healthy way by combining hypnotherapy with exercise and healthy eating, your mind will adjust more easily to losing the initial weight quickly. If you start yoga or a similar exercise routine along with a detox plan, you will lose weight steadily and your body will tone and firm quickly.

How fantastic is that? And what does it ask of you? Two weeks of your time. That is all. If I had a weight problem I would throw myself into a double routine like that tomorrow. I don't have a weight problem, but I still use detox plans because I always feel great during and after them. You have so much more energy when you exercise regularly and feed your body healthy, nutritious food.

Two weeks and a few fruit and vegetable shopping trips are all it takes to galvanize your life in a positive direction. If you want to achieve your weight loss goal badly enough, then start now with a light detox and regular exercise routine. There is nothing as satisfying and rewarding as watching your body become toned and firm. It builds your self-respect and inspires you to live ever more healthily. Once you start you will find that eating very healthily and exercising regularly become a lifestyle. The benefits you will gain from avoiding sugar, sweets, and junk food in general are so rewarding. You will feel so glad when you follow a healthy path and make these changes. Your only regret will be that you didn't start sooner!

Changing Routines and Habits

You need to look at this journey holistically and get rid of anything that holds you back. But to succeed at anything in life that will often be the case. There would be no sense of achievement if it didn't require a little effort along the way. You must shed any unwanted lifestyle habits that may stand in the way of you achieving your goal. Anything that does not help you has to go.

> *If you have a routine that is counterproductive to your goal, make changes.*

If you have a routine that is counterproductive to your goal, make changes. For example, if you enjoy coffee with friends in the morning but doughnuts are also shared, you may need to change this routine. If you can go and avoid the doughnuts then fine, but if the doughnuts are too tempting, avoid this gathering for a while.

If you like to frequent bars and drink alcohol regularly, you'll need to break this habit. Instead of going to a bar, join a gym or tennis club. Or at least balance out the bar excursions with new healthy hobbies. You need to change any routine that is not conducive to losing weight and living healthily and replace it with pursuits that are. Find new activities that you can enjoy and look forward to. With a little determination, you can make changes to your routine that will really help build your motivation.

Developing Your Exercise Plan— and Learning to Enjoy It!

Becoming more active is very important. Do it with a holistic approach that encompasses your everyday life. Simply being more active will help you burn more calories. So each and every day, look for as many ways as possible to become more mobile.

Most of the excuses people make for being overweight are myths. If you eat healthily and exercise regularly, you will become fit and healthy. It is as simple as that. Being big boned or having a slow metabolism is a lame excuse for being overweight. If you sit in front of the TV night after

> "The sovereign invigorator of the body is exercise, and of all the exercises walking is the best."
> —Thomas Jefferson

night and never exercise, you will have a slow metabolism. But if you become more active and exercise often, your metabolism will speed up and you will lose weight more easily. You have the power to choose whether you want a faster or slower metabolism.

To achieve physical fitness, you absolutely must become more active. You can start by simply walking more. It is so easy to drive everywhere these days, but, if you get the opportunity, walk instead. Don't get frustrated if you can't park right outside a restaurant or shop, park a few hundred yards away and walk. Look at the lack of parking spaces as an opportunity to get a little exercise. And, after the meal, the walk back to your car will help you digest your food and burn a few calories.

When you incorporate these ideas into your daily life, they become habits that you get into and enjoy. They also cost you very little time and will become part of your everyday approach to your fitness. Another tip is to avoid escalators and elevators and use the stairs if you can. If you reframe your attitude toward exercise, you will never again be disappointed because an elevator is not working or because you can't find a parking space.

To improve your fitness levels in the long term, you must come from a mind-set that says you are creating a new lifestyle that is holistic and healthy. So many people initially build a strong resolve to get fit only to give up after three months and drift back to their old unhealthy ways. It is a fact that fitness clubs oversell their memberships because 80 percent of people who join them stop going after three months. If all the members of any given gym turned up at once, the gym would not be able to handle the crowd. Think of the tortoise and hare fable, in which the slow but steady pace of the tortoise brings success. Use this story as your metaphor

Work on your fitness gradually by doing a little each day.

for your own long-term success. Work on your fitness gradually by doing a little each day, building up to a level that feels good for you and you are able to maintain.

It can help to find new hobbies and pastimes that fit with your new healthy lifestyle. I highly recommend using yoga, Pilates, or a similar discipline as part of a holistic approach to achieving a weight loss goal. Yoga is a fantastic discipline for toning the body and focusing the mind, and the best way to learn yoga is in a class. If you haven't time to join a class, there are many tutorial DVDs available. The beauty of yoga is that once you learn the basics and a few poses, you can focus on toning specific parts of the body. If yoga is not for you, that's fine. Find other activities that will help you. Swimming, tennis, and badminton are not only good aerobic exercises, but are also enjoyable ways to become more active. Find healthy pursuits that you look forward to and can do regularly to increase your metabolic rate. Aim for some form of exercise every day, even if it is a short, brisk walk.

EXERCISE AND FITNESS OPTIMIZATION TIP

When you get further into your exercise routines, it can help you to find out which type of exercise is best for you to optimize your weight loss. A personal consultation with a qualified fitness coach may help you get the best out of your daily workouts.

As part of my approach to fitness, I find it useful to have a number of exercise aids in and around the house. There is a minitrampoline in my house and a larger one in the garden. Even ten minutes a day bouncing up and down is a great cardiovascular workout that burns calories quickly. This is a fantastic workout because it is quick and easy, and it is a great way to start the day. I can't recommend it highly enough for a daily exercise that you will grow to love.

Go out and buy some weights, a minitrampoline, or a metal frame that can assist with sit-ups. If you don't have the resources or space, then buy an exercise ball. Create a ten-minute workout that you incorporate into your day. The ideal time for this is first thing in the morning—before your morning juice. When you get into regular little exercise routines, your fitness levels will improve, your metabolism will increase, and your desire to improve your fitness will grow even stronger.

TIPS TO QUICK-START A FITNESS ROUTINE

You can get your exercise routine off to a fast start by following these simple tips:

- Avoid any junk food or drinks.
- Stick to three main meals a day and drink lots of fresh water throughout the day.
- Buy a juicer and make yourself fresh juices at least once a day. Use a variety of fruit and vegetables, preferably organic.
- Begin a ten-minute minitrampoline workout first thing each morning, or find another activity that you love and do it daily.
- Be as active as possible throughout your day. Get into the habit of moving your body at every opportunity.
- Empower your mind by using self-hypnosis and/or listening to the CD every day.

Follow these tips for twenty-one days and they will become something you will want to do forever.

Becoming More Active and Loving It

I look forward to my daily workout because I have taught myself to enjoy it. Years ago I would have found it a drag and quit after the initial enthusiasm wore off. Nowadays I am running on a mental program that tells me I love exercise and the rewards it brings. You, too, can reprogram your mind in the same way by using the learning to enjoy exercise technique. When you use self-hypnosis to program your mind to love exercise, you will never again think of it as a struggle. It becomes something that you genuinely enjoy and look forward to every day.

> *Connect exercise with a strong feeling of pleasure and enjoyment.*

The learning to enjoy exercise technique in conjunction with Track 2, "Feel Motivated to Exercise," of the CD will help you to build a strong inner desire to exercise regularly. Stop at this point and read the script through a few times until you are familiar with the technique. The key to getting the most out of this motivational script as well as the CD is to connect exercise with a strong feeling of pleasure and enjoyment. Once you have a grasp of the technique, practice it often so that your desire to exercise and become active on a daily basis is second nature to you.

Learning to Enjoy Exercise Technique

GO TO A quiet darkened room where there are no distractions. Get into a comfortable position, close your eyes, and focus your attention on your breathing. Begin to breathe very slowly and deeply—in through your nose and out through your mouth. Make each breath long and deep; feel your rib cage expand as you breathe in. Continue this for a short while until all the tension disappears from your body and you feel relaxed.

Continue to breathe slowly and deeply in a steady, rhythmical pattern, and when you reach the top of your breath hold it for three seconds: . . . 1 . . . 2 . . . 3. Then silently and mentally count to five on every breath out: . . . 1 . . . 2 . . . 3 . . . 4 . . . 5. Relax more and more with every slow exhale.

Now practice a more instant way of going into a trance. Slowly and steadily count from one to three either silently or out loud: . . . 1 . . . 2 . . . 3. When you reach three, say to yourself, "I will become ten times more deeply relaxed." You will go ten times deeper inside that powerful part of yourself where your true potential resides—your creativity, your courage, and your self-belief. At the very point you reach the number three go deep down into a very relaxed state. So ready? . . . 1 . . . 2 . . . 3. Go there now. More deeply relaxed than you've been in a long time. Every cell in your mind, body, and spirit resonates with positive energy now. Take a short while to connect with this still, centered feeling.

If you don't master this the first time, do not worry because it may take practice before you can go into a deep trance very quickly. If you prefer, you can use one of the other trance-deepening methods described in this book.

Do not be concerned if you feel you are not going very deep. Even if you close your eyes and simply visualize and affirm, you will still make a big difference. The important thing is to do this regularly so that you compound the new images and affirmations. Always remember this: affirmations and visualizations are a remarkably effective reprogramming method *even in the lightest trance states.*

Now to the visualization part. Once you have done the one to three countdown (or whatever deepening method you prefer), begin to create your visualization. Imagine yourself exercising and feel yourself really enjoying it. It is important to use your feelings here so that you anchor a strong sense of enjoyment into your unconscious mind.

Visualize yourself working out at the gym, practicing yoga, playing tennis, cycling, jogging, or doing whatever works for you. As you see yourself doing one or more activities, connect with a feeling of great pleasure and enjoyment. Make the visualization clear, using all five senses to create a realistic mental image. Take a little time to do this, and let your imagination go.

After you have visualized, repeat the following affirmations to yourself in the present tense. With real feeling, say each affirmation ten times or more in a slow, rhythmical way, almost like a slow, steady chant. Imagine every part of you repeating the affirmations with complete conviction and self-belief. Draw the words deep inside you when you say them.

- ➤ I love to exercise and keep fit.
- ➤ I go beyond old limitations and draw out my true potential.
- ➤ I deserve to be fit and healthy.
- ➤ I live my life with courage and self-belief.

These affirmations are examples. Feel free to adapt them for your specific goals. You can even state the affirmations as a soundtrack to your visualization when you get the hang of it.

After you have stated and focused on your affirmations, you can compound these new beliefs by the counting method. Once again, count from one to three. This time, when you reach the number three, affirm that these positive new beliefs will sink ten times deeper into your unconscious mind and that the positive feelings will grow ten times stronger and deeper—into that powerful part of yourself where your true potential lies. So, ready? Slowly count to three: . . . 1 . . . 2 . . . 3, and feel yourself drawing all your new beliefs deep into your inner consciousness. Every aspect of your mind, body, and spirit is resonating with positive energy now. Take a moment to enjoy this feeling and to accept every new belief as a reality.

When you are ready, slowly count from one to ten, open your eyes, and come back to full consciousness.

It is so very important to remain active and to exercise regularly. You absolutely must get into the habit of moving your body and being active on a daily basis so that you are regularly burning calories and maintaining your fitness. Little and often is the key.

The more you move your body each day, the more energy you will have. The combination of healthy diet and regular exercise will help you feel so good that you won't want to go back to your old sluggish ways. The feel-good factor is quite addictive.

By now, you should be well on your way to loving the idea of being more active or at least looking forward to engaging in active pursuits more regularly. Thinking of exercise in this way is a very satisfying and comforting thought. So teach yourself well and see what a wonderful specimen of human determination you can be!

9

Staying Fit
and Healthy for Life

———

*By now, your approach to health and
fitness should have a strong holistic
focus so that every aspect of your life is
geared toward being fit and healthy.*

A FEW years ago, I went on my first and last cruise
vacation. If ever you want to witness overindulgence, a luxury cruise is the place to be. I was amazed at
the food servings. Each meal was five or more courses,
and meals were served at least five times a day. There was
even a midnight buffet, which still attracted the crowds.
It was not a pretty sight to see so many people with so
little control over their eating habits.

The diners in line for the midnight buffet did not need the food, they were simply overindulging. Gluttony had gotten the better of them. Greed is a facet of human nature, and we all have the potential to be greedy. The overindulgence I witnessed turned me off from cruises forever. I now use my freedom of choice to go on vacations that inspire me to be healthier—detoxification, yoga, or fitness retreats, for example. Do whatever feels right for you, but remember that if you mix with people who lack discipline and self-control, these ways may rub off on you. Conversely, healthy, positive people can be inspiring and motivating to be around.

> "A feeble body weakens the mind."
> —Jean Jacques Rousseau

Cutting Back on Excess Will Help You Lose Weight

When people overindulge in one area of their lives, there often are other aspects of their lives that also are out of control. Taking a holistic approach is important, and it is good self-discipline to cut back on yearning and wanting in all areas of your life. Yearning for material things is a waste of energy because it only pushes them away from you. The Tao and other wise teachings tell us that when we don't want anything from anyone or we don't crave material things, we liberate ourselves and become free. Think about that for a moment. There is a freedom and inner peace that comes from letting go of wanting, craving, needing, and yearning. Try it for a few days.

This is a healthy place to aim for because it lightens your mental load. When you live with a nonjudgmental, liberated mind-set, you develop an inner power and you will be attracted toward what you really need. It is your soul's purpose to be healthy, happy, and abundant. So it follows that a healthy discipline to control any tendency toward unnecessary yearning in all areas of your life will also help with your approach to healthy eating.

Maintaining Self-Discipline: Your Body *Is* a Temple

If you owned a car you were fond of, you wouldn't fill it with low-quality gas or not maintain it. You would look after it and figure out how to best optimize its performance. Think of your body in the same way. Well maintained, your body is a magnificent feat of engineering. It will run perfectly if you give it the right fuel. The gift of a healthy body and mind is something

> *Well maintained, your body is a magnificent feat of engineering.*

you should feel a great deal of gratitude for. If you have let your body fall into a little disrepair over the years, the other great gift of life is that you have the ability to repair it to its former glory.

The human body is an amazing thing. It has incredible healing properties, and you can right the wrongs of many years of abuse and neglect when you start to look after it. At the age of seventeen, I contracted hepatitis through alcohol abuse. My excessive drinking from a young age was the result of my unhappy and dysfunctional home life. My doctor at the time ordered me to quit drinking, saying I'd be dead within two years if I didn't. Fortunately, I took his advice. I had to because my liver was severely damaged. It was very scary to be just seventeen and wake up one morning with deep yellow skin and feeling like the life force had been sucked out of my body.

I fully recovered from hepatitis in a few short years, and now in my middle age, I drink occasionally. However, it took me a while to reprogram my thinking and attitude toward alcohol. I had to get rid of the binge drinking mentality I grew up with and teach myself to drink for enjoyment and in moderation.

The amazing thing is that my liver that was once so badly damaged completely repaired itself during my hiatus from alcohol. Isn't it incredible to think that the body is so finely tuned and so wonderfully engineered that it can repair itself? My point is that even if you have abused your body through poor diet, you can make a choice now to put it right. You don't have to keep filling yourself with energy-sapping junk food and drink. Just because so many others live this way, you don't have to. You can choose right now to take back your individuality, break free of that junk food mind-set, and start looking after your greatest assets—your mind and body.

If I am ever in a social situation where everyone is drinking heavily and I don't want to, I simply smile and say that my body is a temple. In the first place, this serves to lightheartedly diffuse the pressure others might put on me to join them in getting drunk. Second, I really mean it. These days my body is a temple, and I can tell you that choosing the healthy option feels so much

> "Start by doing what is necessary, then do what is possible, and suddenly you are doing the impossible."
>
> —St. Francis of Assisi

more comforting and satisfying than to be stuck in a boozing, smoking, junk-food-eating lifestyle. That was my past life; I will never go back. These days I wake up in the mornings with so much more energy. I generally feel brighter, fitter, and healthier in so many ways that the thought of my old lifestyle fills me with dread and horror. The benefits I feel from consistently eating healthy, high-quality food and avoiding junk food and drink are awesome. My only regret is that I wish I had known this when I was young. But, life is all about experience and learning.

Just recently, after a business meeting, someone gave me a box of chocolates. I accepted graciously, knowing I would not keep them. However, it made me think, *Why do we more often give each other unhealthy food as a gift than healthy food? Why at Easter when we are celebrating a religious event do we overdose our children on chocolate and candy?*

The thing to remember is you don't have to run with the pack or follow herd mentality. Just because everyone else eats candy two or three times a week, goes boozing on weekends, or drinks coffee every morning, you don't have to. Just because everyone else allows their children to consume tons of chocolate at Easter or stuff themselves silly at Christmas, you don't have to. Think for yourself. Because everyone else is doing something and it seems the norm, it doesn't necessarily mean it is a good thing.

> *You don't have to run with the pack or follow herd mentality.*

Immersing Yourself in Your New Healthy Lifestyle

By now, your approach to health and fitness should have a strong holistic focus so that every aspect of your life is geared toward being fit and healthy. You will succeed if you make lots of small positive changes in your life that collectively give you a powerful drive to reach your target weight. So continue to make as many large and small changes as you can that are congruent with your goal.

It can also help if you focus on personal goals that allow you to fulfill your potential. Think of opportunities to be more creative and new ways in which you can express your inner talents. The CD and self-hypnosis techniques in this book will help you tap into your creative talents. Think of new hobbies that you would like to develop that will contribute to your healthy lifestyle. Do you like reading, writing, painting, singing, or dancing? Make your goals big and bold. Maybe you want to travel more. You might want to swim in the Red Sea, fly over the Grand Canyon, visit the Taj Mahal or the Pyramids of Giza, or see the Great Barrier Reef. Whatever your life goals, set your sights on achieving them now.

> *You will succeed if you make lots of small positive changes in your life that collectively give you a powerful drive to reach your target weight.*

Making positive changes in all areas of your life will help your overall approach to weight and fitness. Here are some examples of positive changes. Read them and then make your own list.

- Make a habit of reading self-improvement books.
- Watch DVDs that educate and inspire you.
- Travel to different places—list the places you want to visit.
- Learn to play a musical instrument.
- Start your own business.
- Join a meditation or an inspirational group with others who have positive aspirations.
- Take up a new skill that will help you in some way—learn a language, go horseback riding, study graphology, and so on. The possibilities are endless.

There are a million and one opportunities today to improve our lives. You will enrich your life when you go forward, learn new things, and educate yourself. By filling your days with positive pursuits and making plans, you will no longer focus on food. Your food intake should be three healthy meals a day, and you should only think about each meal at the time you eat it. Instead, focus your thoughts on the day ahead and what you are going to achieve that day.

> "Twenty years from now you will be more disappointed by the things that you didn't do than by the ones you did do."
>
> —Mark Twain

Make a list of life goals that you want to achieve. The first goals must include reaching your target weight and achieving lasting fitness. Then include other life goals that support your new healthy lifestyle.

Write a list of life goals below and include a time frame for each (if relevant).

Review these goals every six months, adding to or adapting them each time so they remain fresh. Post your goals in places, such as your bathroom, office, or car, where you will read them daily. By giving your goals this daily focus, you will be amazed at how many of these things you will have achieved after six months.

Making plans and setting clear goals for your future are important. When you do these things, you will get a sense of purpose and direction. They also help you maintain a positive outlook. This is important because being stuck in a negative rut or feeling depressed can lead to overeating and a lack of motivation to look after your health. You can avoid this trap by filling your life with as many positive things as possible.

It's Your Choice

When you learn to harness your inner energy, you will achieve your weight loss goal. With the right will and determination, you have the potential to dramatically improve the quality of your life. So what are you waiting for? Make the simple choice to look after yourself. The rewards are great. When you get into the habit of empowering your mind and energizing your body, your health and well-being will improve in so many ways. When your mind is positive and your body healthy, your aura also will be strong and healthy. Many metaphysicians believe illnesses start in the aura before manifesting in the physical body.

> *With the right will and determination, you have the potential to dramatically improve the quality of your life.*

It is so comforting and satisfying to feel fit and healthy and in control of your eating habits. It is also an easy decision to make; you just need to keep your focus and concentration. To achieve anything in life will require a little discipline and self-control. Whether you want to be a sportsman, own your own business, or lose weight, you need discipline and self-control. It is the same for any goal you set for yourself. Whatever you want, don't expect it to fall into your lap or look to others to give it to you. Nobody owes you anything, *you* have to go out there and make it happen.

If you ever need inspiration, watch the athletes who compete in the Paralympics for those with physical disabilities. In spite of their disabilities, they achieve their sporting goals through sheer determination and hard work. Watch them power toward the finish line in a big race, knowing all their hard work and efforts have been for that moment. To focus all of your energy into being the best in a sport when you are disabled takes huge courage and self-belief. But that courage and self-belief is something we all have when we become disciplined and focused. You, too, possess great determination and resolve, and by now you will be using that energy to power toward achieving your goal to become fit and healthy.

> *It is so comforting and satisfying to feel fit and healthy and in control of your eating habits. It is also an easy decision to make; you just need to keep your focus and concentration.*

Now that you have read through the book, used the self-hypnosis techniques, and listened to the CD a few times, say to yourself, "I deserve to be fit and healthy and in good shape." How does that feel? Now that you have absorbed the contents of this book and CD, it will feel like an absolute truth!

Checklist of Key Habits to Cultivate

Read through this list regularly to see if you are following these guidelines.

- ❑ Visualize yourself at your ideal target weight regularly and believe it is a reality.

- ❑ Repeat your affirmations daily.

- ❑ Focus on your self-hypnosis techniques and listen to the CD regularly.

- ❑ Free yourself from any bad habits or negative conditioning.

- ❑ Do not weigh yourself or use the word *diet*. Do not discuss your weight with anyone. Maintain a ⸱nt, disciplined quest to improve the quality of ⸱ life.

❑ Stick to three small, healthy main meals a day— breakfast, lunch, and dinner. Avoid eating late.

❑ Avoid processed food and food with excess sugar, additives, or chemicals. Choose organic food whenever possible.

❑ Drink fresh mineral water (that you love the taste of) between meals in place of snacking.

❑ Always eat very slowly, chew your food thoroughly, and be fully engaged in the process of eating. Stop eating as soon as you are full.

❑ Be grateful for each healthy meal.

❑ Get into the habit of moving your body as often as possible. Look for simple everyday opportunities to be active.

❑ Exercise little and often, every day if possible, even if it is just a short walk or a minitrampoline workout for ten minutes in the morning.

❑ Never criticize yourself, and apply the 80/20 rule from Chapter 7.

❑ Regularly program your mind to love your new healthy, holistic lifestyle.

Finally

My goal has been to help you create a holistic approach to achieving weight loss and lasting fitness by using many small building blocks and a few major therapy techniques. By now you should have embraced many changes and be well on your way to achieving your weight loss goal. I sincerely hope that is the case. This whole journey must be something you really enjoy, and your positive approach to food and exercise must become second nature to you. That must be your ultimate aim. If you learn to love being fit and healthy, everything else will fall into place. I have adopted these methods myself, and avoiding junk food and sweets is now second nature to me. I also have a powerful inner desire to exercise regularly. These positive habits get stronger all the time simply because of my inner programming.

When you work on your affirmations, use the techniques, and listen to the CD regularly, this will become your reality. You will develop a core belief that you love being healthy and in good shape. I suggest you continue to use all of these tools to make that belief as strong as possible . . . so that you pride yourself on having the discipline you need to remain fit and healthy . . . so that you find it easy to say no to chocolate, desserts, or fattening foods that are no good for you . . . so that you regularly look for opportunities to exercise and enjoy the feeling you get from it.

When you are at this point, you will be in complete control of your weight and fitness, and it will feel so satisfying and comforting to you. In fact, you will wonder how you ever felt any different. So keep immersing your inner mind with positive programming and you will achieve your goals.

I wish you every success.

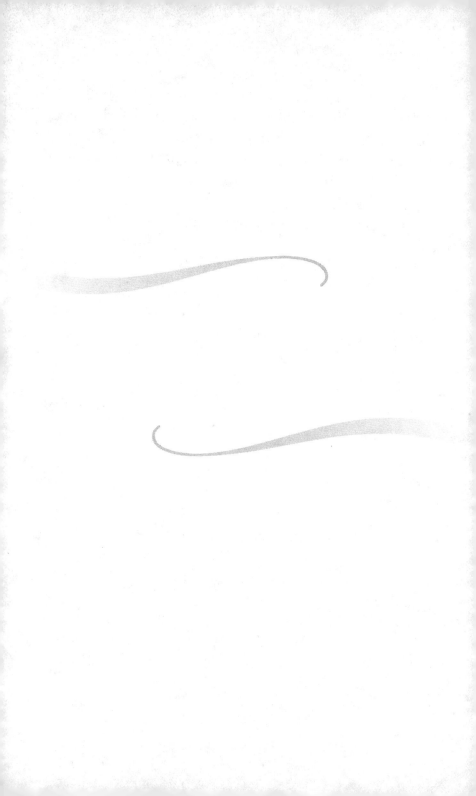

CD Guidelines

THE HYPNOTHERAPY CD that accompanies this book is completely safe and very effective, and it comes with a clear set of instructions. It has two tracks. Track 1, "Lose Weight Now," is a thirty-three-minute hypno-therapy session that will help you to eat healthily, build your self-esteem, and reach your target weight. Track 2, "Feel Motivated to Exercise," is a thirty-minute hypno-therapy session that will help you build the motivation to exercise and keep fit.

You can use both tracks repeatedly, or focus on one track if you need more attention in a particular area. There are no rules, but I do recommend that in the early stages you listen to either one or both tracks on the CD at least once a day.

You must never listen to the CD while driving a vehi-cle or using heavy machinery. The recordings on this CD will guide you into a state of complete physical and mental relaxation, so it is recommended that you listen while lying down in a place where you won't be disturbed. For maximum effect, it is strongly recommended that you listen through headphones. When listening to either track, make sure you listen all the way through without interruptions.

Don't worry if you fall asleep before you reach the end of a track. Your unconscious mind is very capable of absorbing all the positive suggestions even during light sleep states.

CD Contents

———

THERE ARE five stages to each hypnotherapy session on the CD:

1. Introduction
2. Induction
3. Trance deepening
4. Posthypnotic suggestions and affirmations
5. Awakening

Stage 1: Introduction

The first thing you will hear is the introductory music and an explanation of how the CD works. After a few minutes the music fades and you are left with a pleasant voice and some uniquely created sound effects that will guide you into a state of complete physical and mental relaxation. Some of the sound effects have been recorded at sixty beats per minute to help synchronize the left and right hemispheres of the brain and create a very receptive learning state. The sounds are also recorded in certain keys and at frequencies that induce positive feelings.

Stage 2: Induction

The induction is the first stage of trance, created via breathing techniques and by using exercises that release tension and stress.

Stage 3: Trance Deepening

This stage is the guiding down into a deeper state of hypnosis. It can be achieved by counting down from ten to one or via many other deepening techniques. Once in a deeper state of hypnosis, the listener is more receptive to suggestion.

Stage 4: Posthypnotic Suggestions and Affirmations

On each hypnotherapy session you will hear echoed affirmations that pan slowly from left to right in your speakers or headphones. This relaxing and unique effect is very hypnotic and helps you to absorb each affirmation deeply. In this receptive and relaxed state, you will also be given a number of positive posthypnotic suggestions to help you achieve your weight loss goal.

Posthypnotic suggestions are the most important stage of the process because these empower, motivate, dispel fears, and have a powerful, lasting effect. The posthypnotic suggestions given to the listener when in a deeply relaxed and receptive state will be acted upon at a later date. For example, a hypnotherapist may make a posthypnotic suggestion such as "I love to exercise and keep fit." When you are deeply relaxed these affirmations help to reprogram your thoughts, and you will then respond to these suggestions automatically in your daily life. The motivation to exercise and keep fit then becomes normal and natural—something you love doing. The key is to draw the affirmations deep inside you and really believe with every fiber and cell in your mind and body that they are a reality. The more energy you give the affirmations, the stronger the belief becomes.

Affirmations work in a way similar to posthypnotic suggestions. They are first-person, present-tense phrases that you will affirm to yourself as a reality now. For example, "I feel confident and secure."

Stage 5: Awakening

The awakening is the gentle transgression from deep relaxation and alpha-state consciousness to full, waking

consciousness. This can be achieved by using posthypnotic suggestions and a slow count up from one to ten.

The important thing to remember when using the
CD is that although you are being guided, you will always remain in full control of the whole process. If at any
time you need to awaken, you just open your eyes and
you will be wide awake.

Track 1: "Lose Weight Now"

This track is a thirty-three-minute hypnotherapy session to help you eat healthily, build your self-esteem, and
reach your target weight. Affirmations and subliminal
suggestions include:

- I am in complete control of my eating habits.
- I love the taste of pure fresh water.
- I remain a healthy eater forever.
- My self-esteem grows stronger and stronger.
- I love to exercise regularly and keep fit.
- I deserve to be fit and healthy.

Track 2: "Feel Motivated to Exercise"

Track 2 is a thirty-minute hypnotherapy session to help
you to build a powerful motivation to exercise and keep
fit. Affirmations and subliminal suggestions include:

- I love to exercise and keep fit.
- I go beyond old limitations and draw out my true potential.
- I deserve to be fit and healthy.
- I live my life to the fullest with courage and self-belief.

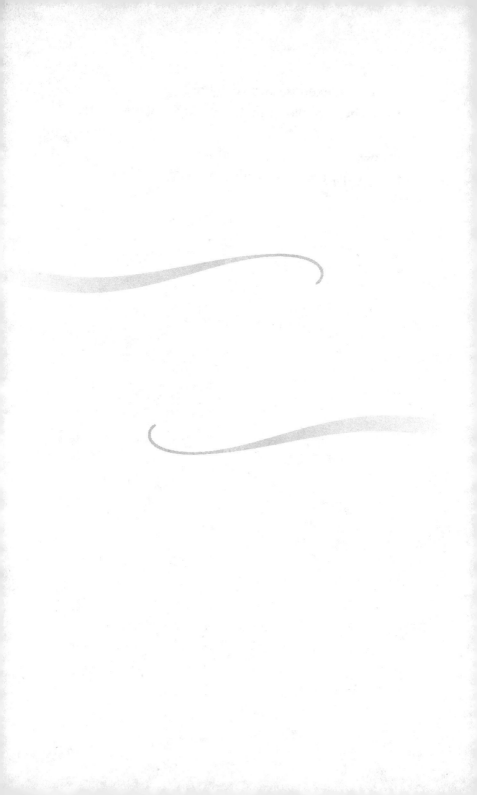

Resources

Books

Elman, Dave. *Hypnotherapy* (Westwood Publishing Company, 1984). A classic on hypnosis first published in 1960 and still very relevant.

Grace, Janey Lee. *Imperfectly Natural Woman: Getting Life Right the Natural Way* (Crown House Publishing, 2005). A fabulous book on holistic living from a writer with a grounded approach.

Holford, Patrick. *New Optimum Nutrition Bible: The Book You Have to Read if You Care About Your Health* (Piatkus Books, 2004). This explains how, by giving yourself the best possible intake of nutrients, to allow your body to be as healthy as it possibly can be.

Lawrence, Felicity. *Not on the Label* (E-Penguin General, 2004). An eye-opening book on the food industry. A must read!

Vale, Jason. *Chocolate Busters: The Easy Way to Kick Your Addiction* (HarperCollins, 2005). Will help you break the chocolate habit forever.

Vale, Jason. *The Juice Master: Turbo-Charge Your Life in 14 Days* (HarperCollins, 2005). Commonsense advice on healthy eating with many valuable tips. Includes an excellent detox plan.

DVDs

Byrne, Rhonda, Paul Harrington, Michael Beckwith, and Neale Donald Walsch. *The Secret* (extended edition; TS Productions, 2007). Philosophers, metaphysicians, and quantum physicists discuss the universal law of attraction and demonstrate how your inner thoughts create your outer reality.

Harrold, Glenn. *Lose Weight Now* (Diviniti Publishing, 2007). A forty-minute lose-weight hypnotherapy DVD that includes subliminal imagery.

Rea, Shiva. *Yoga Shakti* (Gemini Sun, 2004). A professional DVD for a complete yoga workout.

Vale, Jason. *The Juicemaster's Rebounding Workout* (Juicemaster, 2007). Everything you need to know about working out on a minitrampoline.

CDs and Audiotapes

Harrold, Glenn. *Build Your Self-Esteem* (Diviniti Publishing, 2002). A high-quality hypnotherapy CD that will help you build strong self-esteem.

Harrold, Glenn. *Lose Weight Now* (Diviniti Publishing, 2002). A high-quality hypnotherapy CD to help you release any need or desire for sweet, fattening food and feel good about eating smaller amounts of healthy food.

Harrold, Glenn. *Overcome Addictions* (Diviniti Publishing, 2005). A high-quality hypnotherapy CD that will help you release any type of addiction, including food, alcohol, gambling, drugs, TV, Internet, sex, computers, shopping, nicotine, caffeine, dieting, chocolate, nail biting, and work.

Harrold, Glenn. *Unleash Your True Potential* (Diviniti Publishing, 2003). A superb high-quality hypnosis CD combining skilled hypnotherapy techniques with state-of-the-art digital recording technology.

Index